THE THEORY OF BINOCULAR VISION

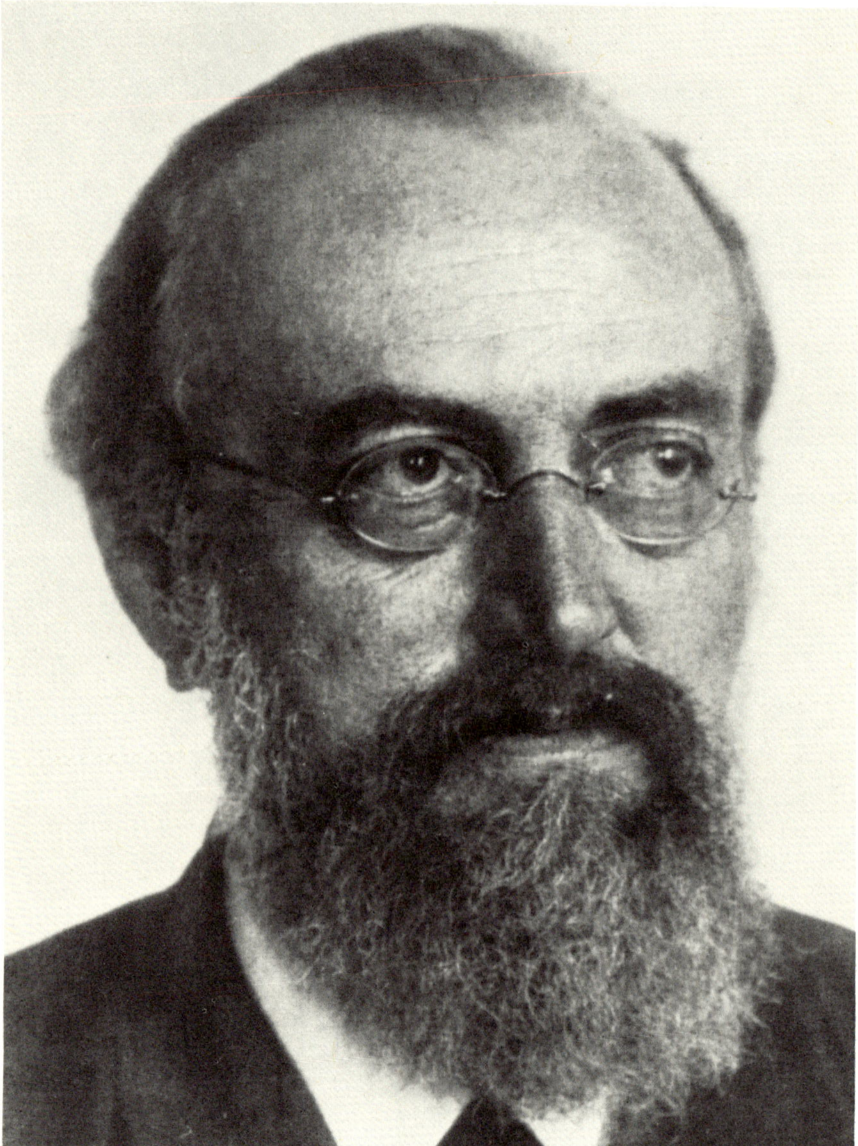

Ewald Hering

THE THEORY OF BINOCULAR VISION

Ewald Hering (1868)

Edited by
Bruce Bridgeman
University of California, Santa Cruz
and
Lawrence Stark
University of California, Berkeley

Translation and Introduction by
Bruce Bridgeman
Commentary by
Lawrence Stark

PLENUM PRESS · NEW YORK AND LONDON

Library of Congress Cataloging in Publication Data

Hering, Ewald, 1834-1918.
The theory of binocular vision.

Translation of Die Lehre vom binokularen Sehen.
Includes bibliographical references and index.
1. Binocular vision. I. Bridgeman, Bruce. II. Stark, Lawrence. III. Title.
[DNLM: 1. Vision. WW400 H546L]
QP487.H413 1977 612'.846 76-30836
ISBN 0-306-31016-3

The German text, underlying the present translation is *Die Lehre vom Binokularen Sehen*, by Ewald Hering, published by Wilhelm Englemann in Leipzig in 1868.

A Division of Plenum Publishing Corporation
227 West 17th Street, New York, N.Y. 10011

Printed in the United States of America

Contents

Part Three

On the Eye Muscles

Part Four

On the Accommodation of the Double Eye

Introduction

The Theory of Binocular Vision is a book about neurological control theory. In this sense it was far ahead of its time, for the formal development of control theory was many decades in the future when this book appeared in 1868. Hering's principal concept is that the control of eye movements is greatly simplified if there is only *one* neurological control system commanding the 'double-eye' as a single organ. This idea leads directly to the first thorough exposition of what is now known as Hering's law, that the corresponding muscles of the two eyes are always equally innervated. As Hering eloquently states it, "one and the same impulse of will directs both eyes simultaneously as one can direct a pair of horses with single reins" (Ch. 2).

The 19th Century

The book was written during an exciting era for physiological research. Before the mid-19th century the study of physiology had been limited to isolated efforts by great men who worked largely without colleagues or organized laboratories. Now for the first time sensory physiology was becoming a living field of inquiry, with many groups working simultaneously on fundamental problems. Like the classical Greeks before them in philosophy, the physiologists of the 19th century were defining in a burst of creative energy the problems which would shape subsequent inquiry; and like the Greeks, they produced a splendid period of science.

A period of a few decades in the middle of the 19th century yielded many of the principles which have now come to be taken for granted as axioms of biological science. Though the existence of cells was known before the 1840's, for instance, many biologists thought that much of living matter in higher organisms was organized as tissues rather than as aggregates of cells. Advances in microscopy made it possible for Schwann and Schleiden to firmly establish cell theory in the 1840's as a basis of biology, but the independent existence of nerve cells with continuous membranes was not completely accepted until near the turn of the 20th century (see Coleman, 1971). Even such a fundamental concept as the conservation of energy was not stated clearly until 1847, when Helmholtz introduced it in a physiological context. Within a single lifetime, study of the processes of life was transformed from a branch of idealist *Naturphilosophie* into a rigorous science much like the one we know today.

One of the founders of this new experimental physiology was Johannes Müller, whose 1840 *Handbook of Physiology* greatly influenced Hering. Although Müller considered himself to be a nativist rather than an empiricist, emphasizing inherited organizations over learned ones, that did not mean that he was not a capable experimenter. Today it is easy to identify empiricists with the experimental tradition at the expense of the nativists; by the mid-ninteenth century, however, both groups were committed to the experimental method developed by the physical sciences. But Müller believed in vitalism, while most of the generation following him was convinced that only the common physical and chemical forces were active within the organism. They shared the conviction that only mechanistic, reductionistic inquiry could uncover the mysteries of the living organism, and they opposed the vitalists who still insisted on the unknowable nature of the spark of life. It was this new mechanistic outlook which made experimental physiology in the modern sense possible, and the fact that a philosophical position was at the bottom of the scientific effort emphasizes the important role which a philosophy can play in the development of a science.

The new mechanistic feeling was more than just a vague change of intellectual emphasis; while still in their twenties, four of Müller's students, all later to become famous physiologists, explicitly agreed on a pact to root out vitalism (Cranefield, 1957). In order of age they were Carl Ludwig, Emil du Bois-Reymond, Ernst Brücke, and Hermann von Helmholtz. The year was 1847.

The movement to reduce physiology to physics and chemistry was a vigorous but brief one, lasting roughly from the pact of 1847 to the 1870's, and it exhausted itself simply because the task could be accomplished in a few decades given the relatively undeveloped state of the disciplines at that time and the genius of the men who devoted themselves to the problem (Cranefield, 1957). The present book is a part of that effort. After the movement had redefined the direction of the life sciences it found itself without adequate knowledge either of physical sciences or of physiology to progress much further, so that the focus returned to gathering data within the disciplines.

At this time physiological optics was at the frontier of the investigation of mechanistic bases of perception. Psychology was yet to become independent of philosophy and physiology, and what we would call experimental and physiological psychology today were still part of physiology (Boring, 1950). So Hering, Helmholtz, and their colleagues were extending themselves as far as anyone could into the investigation of physiological mechanisms of experience. *The Theory of Binocular Vision* was written very much with this feeling of the unity of physiological and psychological inquiry; it was part of Hering's task to show how the nature of eye movements reflects not only the kinematics of the eye but also the visual perceptions of the observer. ". . . The motor apparatus of the visual organ must match its sensory apparatus as the shell does the egg" (Ch. 19).

The new experimental physiology produced a group of intelligent and creative men so large that it cannot be explained by chance alone; the *Zeitgeist* (spirit or mood of the times) must have had an influence as well. Donders, Listing, Weber and Fechner were all active at this time. Now each name defines a "law" of vision or psychophysics. Mach, Meissner, Wundt, and many others were also already engaged in pioneering work. But the giant among them was Hermann von Helmholtz, whose monumental three-volume *Physiological Optics* (1867) defined the field for decades to come.

Hering's Early Career

It was into this milieu that Ewald Hering came. Born in Altgersdorf in southern Prussia in 1834, he grew up in his father's parsonage in a country environment. His early love of nature led eventually to the study of medicine at Leipzig, from 1853 to 1858. There he was taught by E.H. Weber, G.T. Fechner, O. Funke, and by J.V. Carus, with whom he journeyed to the Gulf of Messina to study annelids in the winter semester of 1858-9 (Garten, 1918). None of these mentors had as strong an influence during this time, however, as Müller: Hering later called himself "an enthusiastic, if not direct, student of Johannes Müller" (Hering, 1884).

From 1860 to 1865 Hering remained in Leipzig as a practicing physician and clinical assistant while writing his first major work, the five-volume *Beiträge zur Physiologie (Contributions to Physiology)* (1861-1864), which was devoted to problems of visual space perception. In these volumes he attacked the empiricism of Helmholtz and Wundt on many grounds and supported his own ideas with careful reasoning and experimental observations. Helmholtz recognized the importance of the work by devoting large sections of the final volume of his *Physiological Optics* to critiques of it. While the first works of many researchers lack sophistication in the handling of difficult questions, Hering's *Beiträge* established his reputation almost immediately, leading to his appointment as professor of physiology and medical physics at the Josephsakademie in Vienna. Though the Josephsakademie was intended to train doctors for the Austro-Hungarian military and had little patience with other activities, Hering still found time for research.

The Hering-Helmholtz Controversies

Hering must have reacted strongly to Volume III of Helmholtz's *Physiological Optics* (1866). Helmholtz's complete work was published in 1867, and *The Theory of Binocular Vision* appeared in the following year with an extensive critique of Helmholtz and a radically simple view of the nature of eye movements. The young professor attacked with considerable courage, for when *Physiological Optics* appeared he was 32 years old and just beginning his first post, while Helmholtz, 45, was already held in awe by the scientific community.

The controversy between Hering and Helmholtz, which continued for decades on many fronts, is almost the classic example of a fruitful scientific rivalry. The conflict of their opinions is deceptive, however, for the two could hold polar-opposite views on some issues only because they defined and approached the fundamental problems of physiology in the same way. Both were mechanists who spent considerable energy in the successful struggle against vitalism, and both shared a respect for careful experiments and observations, even when performed by an opponent. They actually agreed in a wide range of potentially controversial areas, for instance in the 'outflow' theory of visual localization and in the kinematics of eye positions. Their extensive reviews of one another's work, and even their painstaking critiques of one another, show their mutual respect. It is their disagreements, however, which have received the most attention, and these sometimes grew quite heated. Each had the habit of referring to the parts of the other's work with which he agreed as 'discoveries,' while disputed parts were sarcastically labelled 'announcements,' 'declarations,' or worse.

In *The Theory of Binocular Vision* Hering developed the law bearing his name, which states simply that the two eyes share a common innervation. Neither eye can be moved without the other being affected in some way. This may seem obvious even to a casual observer, but Helmholtz was not a casual observer. In his *Physiological Optics* he asserted at some length that each eye could be moved independently, and that the two eyes came to be used together only by habit in the interest of single clear vision. This opinion was a necessary corollary of Helmholtz's thoroughgoing empiricism, assigning as little as possible to inborn abilities. Helmholtz countered Hering's (and Müller's) assertion of inborn coordination between the two eyes by pointing out numerous cases where the two eyes seem to move independently, or where one moves while the other remains fixed. Examples of such seemingly independent movements include those made during asymmetrical vergence, where an object moves toward the observer along the line of sight of one eye so that only the other eye must move to maintain binocular fixation. Helmholtz also describes small prism-induced vertical movements of one eye while the other remains fixed, and "cyclofusional" movements of one eye made to track an image as it tilts on the retina.

Such examples forced Hering to produce in *The Theory of Binocular Vision* a more sophisticated account of the coordination of the eyes. His many experiments and observations resulted in several proofs of Hering's law, some of them since neglected. The observations include studies of movements of occluded, suppressed, or blinded eyes; movements of *both* eyes during asymmetrical vergence; eye coordinations in newborns; maintenance of coordination in cases of eye muscle paresis; and binocular coordination during nystagmus. None of these types of movement aid vision, and some hinder it, so that their existence constitutes for Hering a powerful set of proofs of the inborn coordination of the eyes. Hering also goes beyond negative reactions to Helmholtz in proving the innervation law by several independent methods, and in providing other reasons why such a law would aid the control of eye movements. But it is best to let the text speak for itself on these matters.

Though Hering's approach has been summarized in the word

'nativism,' he explicitly rejected that label (Hillebrand, 1918), and even early in his career he had to complain that ". . . My opinion has been caricatured as though I let the child into the light of the world already completely educated as a visual virtuoso, and as though the images of external objects were shoved from the eye onto the stage of consciousness fully complete in form and color like sets from the wings of a theater" (Ch. 23). Hering attacked the excesses of the empiricism of his day while tempering nativism with a surprisingly modern view of the close coordination (one might almost say the inborn coordination) between genetically and environmentally derived organizations of the sensory apparatus. So his view was surprisingly close to the modern one that information from the genes and information from the environment combine in every action. Unlike Kant, who used pure philosophical reasoning to arrive at *a priori* ideas of space and time, Hering based his modified nativism on careful and well-controlled experiment. This may explain why Hering never referred directly to Kant in explaining his philosophical position.

The Twentieth Century

What was the outcome of these century-old nature-nuture controversies? Many of them are still alive. Disputes over the origin and nature of differences in intellectual ability, for instance, continue unabated, with the same misconceptions being advanced in the twentieth century as were aired in the nineteenth. Although Helmholtz enjoyed enormous prestige during his lifetime, the consensus now favors Hering on many issues, including those relating to Hering's law. (One reason for Helmholtz's great prestige in the English-speaking world may be that his *Physiological Optics* has been translated, while until now the immediate response of his leading contemporary critic has not.) Even in the appendix to the 1925 English edition of Helmholtz's *Physiological Optics* there is a statement by Professor von Kries that "the ocular muscles cannot act except in perfectly definite combinations, all other combinations being impossible" (p. 625). Hering's ideas also prevailed in the method of definition of the axes of eye movements, where modern practice follows the conventions of Ch. 13. It must be said that Helmholtz's work in large part founded the modern field of physiological optics, and that many of his mathematical feats have not been bettered. His extremist empiricism is now dead, however, and a century of subsequent work has revealed an extensive inherited structure of behavior which follows the same rules as the inheritance of the structures of anatomy. The two interact in sometimes subtle ways in the development of the visual system (reviewed by Blakemore, 1973; Pribram & Bridgeman, 1976), with the environment acting to 'tune' the genetically determined mechanism for optimal function. But as Hering notes in his book, the tuning is possible only within narrowly defined limits.

The Theory of Binocular Vision is useful today scientifically as well as historically, partly because physiological optics has made relatively little progress beyond what was accomplished in the 1860's. One current value of the book is instructional, for Hering's conception of eye movement control is astonishingly simple at its base. First, the double eye concept greatly simplifies thinking about eye movements. The complex actions of the twelve eye muscles (described here in Fig. 26, though usually credited to Hering in 1879) are resolved into three binocular motors corresponding to the three coordinates of Cartesian space, and the innervations of the motors are independent of the starting point of the movement. Listing's and Donders' laws follow from this conception, becoming indirect corollaries of a complete statement of Hering's law. These principles apply within the 'smaller fixation space,' the range in which people ordinarily make eye movements without supplementary head movements. Hering discusses deviations from this basic conception only after it is established both theoretically and experimentally. From a contemporary point of view the only gross inaccuracies in the book are those dealing with the dynamics of eye movement, for saccadic eye movements had not yet been differentiated from pursuit movements when the book was written. In fact it is surprising how much Hering and his contemporaries could do without the availability of objective methods of measuring eye movements.

But there is another side to the book. Hering was out of step with his contemporaries in much of his thinking, and Hurvich (1969) cites several accurate observations for which Hering was vilified by his colleagues. One of them centered around the description of the cellular structure of the liver, where Hering described the blood flow in one way, through small round tubules, while the most influential physiologists of his time (Pflüger in Germany and Beale in Britain) described it in quite another way. Hering's opponents prevailed until Hans Elias (1949), while preparing laboratory teaching materials for medical students, discovered to his surprise that the establishment had been wrong and that Hering had been correct. Another example of Hering's defeat and posthumous vindication originates in this book; the controversy concerns cyclofusional movements of the eyes.

Cyclofusion – An Example

In addition to movements of the line of sight, the eyes can execute rotations about the line of sight as an axis. The iris rotates like a wheel, with the line of sight as the axle. In the current translation this type of motion has been given the modern label of 'cyclorotation'; Hering considered it to be of primary importance, listing it among the three kinds of eye movements in the first paragraph of this book. According to Wundt (1862), all early study of eye movements was devoted to this kind of movement. With the head fixed, the issue is whether the two eyes can execute simultaneous cyclorotations in opposite directions, one clockwise and the other counterclockwise. These are called 'cyclofusional movements' in the older literature because their sole visual function is the fusion of images which are rotated against one another. A more unambiguous modern label is 'disjunctive cyclorotations.'

Hering asserts in Ch. 14 that such movements do not occur, and gives experimental proofs to support his stand. Aware that most of his contemporaries believed in the existence of disjunctive cyclorotation, he also describes the experiment which led them to that conclusion, using as a stimulus the rotation of two identical images against one another in a stereoscope. Fusion can be maintained if the rotation is small, proving to the satisfaction of most physiologists that disjunctive cyclorotational movements had occurred. But Hering was not so quick to draw any conclusions, and he did one additional control experiment. Instead of using an image consisting of only one vertical line in each half of the stereoscope, he drew two parallel lines for each image (Fig. 11). Then it was a simple matter to fuse the more medial of the two lines in each image so that three lines were visible: the center line would be seen binocularly while each of the lines flanking it would be seen with only one eye. Hering then tilted both cards in the stereoscope so that their tops moved inward toward one another; the binocular center line remained fused while the two flanking lines tilted. This showed that the continued fusion was a result of our ability to fuse two images which lie on slightly different retinal locations (within Panum's fusional area). (This experiment is so simple and the results so dramatic that I have used it sucessfully as a classroom demonstration.)

Hering follows this demonstration with another experiment contradicting the importance of disjunctive cyclorotations, this time using complex stimuli. Two identical images are rotated against one another in a stereoscope and are again fused; when fusion is broken by separating the images or by gently shaking them while holding a prominent vertical contour of the image in the eye, the doubled contour has the divergence which was noted at the beginning of the experiment. Alternatively one can begin rotating the images after they have been fused; when the rotation becomes so large that fusion breaks, the images instead of rotating away from one another immediately show a rotational disparity which cannot be resolved by voluntary disjunctive cyclorotations.

In the century since the publication of these experiments the difference between cyclofusion and cyclorotation seems to have been forgotten or ignored by many workers who equated the ability to fuse two rotated stimuli with the ability to make an equally large disjunctive cyclorotation (i.e., Hofmann and Bielchowsky (1900), Brecher (1934), Verhoeff (1934.) Alpern reviewed most of this literature in 1962, noting Hering's claim in *The Theory of Binocular Vision* that such movements do not occur, but the parallel-line experiment described above was not reviewed. Ogle included a whole chapter on disjunctive cyclorotations, including new experiments, in his book on binocular vision (1964) without citing Hering's 1868 book. Hering's opinion appeared to be dead and buried in the literature.

Recently the issue has been re-examined with objective methods of measuring cyclorotations. Kertesz and Jones (1970) measured the movements by automatically scanning an appropriately marked contact lens fitting tightly on a subject's eye; they found no evidence of disjunctive cyclorotation, though the subjects could fuse rotationally disparate vertical lines. Kertesz (1972) later repeated and extended these observations in another laboratory. Crone and Everhard-Halm (1975), however, claim to have found disjunctive cyclorotations using a photographic method, noting that Kertesz and Jones (1970) had used stimuli which would not be expected to elicit the movements. Crone and Everhard-Halm also note that subjective and objective methods give closely similar results if the subjective method involves aligning two monocular stimuli which are distinct from the fused image; this is the method which Hering used in the parallel-line experiment. (In 1879, speaking of himself in the third person, Hering recanted his earlier position and noted that disjunctive cyclorotations can occur under some conditions.) The modern view of the controversy is that cyclofusion is the result of a complex combination of cyclorotation and the psychological rotational fusion which we might call 'Hering fusion.' The relative contribution of each mechanism depends upon the complexity of the stimulus, the orientations of its features, and the degree of rotation, interacting in ways which still are not clearly understood. In this case as in others the truth seems to lie somewhere between the stands of the earlier antagonists: if disjunctive cyclorotations do exist, they do not necessarily correspond to the degree of rotation of fused monocular images. In short, modern workers have rediscovered the hard way that cyclorotation and cyclofusion are distinct and separable.

Hering's Subsequent Career

After writing *The Theory of Binocular Vision* Hering went on to a long and productive career in physiology. Partly as a result of this book he was called to succeed Purkinje at Prague, where he spent 25 years as head of an active institute studying color vision and spatial aspects of vision, and later pioneering in the new science of electrophysiology. He also served for many years as Rector of the German university in Prague. Twice Hering's name was put forward for a professorship in physiology in Vienna, and both times the selection committee was in his favor. The appointment was blocked both times by Brücke, a staunch ally of Helmholtz, who never trusted Hering. So for most of his professional life Hering remained an outsider in two ways, as a German in a Czech city and as a frequent intellectual opponent of Helmholtz and the scientific establishment of the time.

Hering's principal work in vision during this period is summarized in his *Zur Lehre vom Lichtsinn (Toward a Theory of the Light Sense)* (1878) and *Der Raumsinn und die Bewegungen des Auges (Spatial Sense and Movements of the Eye)* (1879). During this period he developed another contradiction of Helmholtz in his famous opponent-processes theory of color vision. Hints of its early development appear in this book (Ch. 15). Helmholtz subscribed to the theory of Newton and of Young that the color sense was based on three primary colors which combine in various ways to yield all color sensations. Hering described color perception in terms of opponent processes; red was not only different from green, but its opposite. The same applied to yellow and blue, and to light and dark. Each side had strong data and arguments, and again the two views seemed irreconcilable. As usual Helmholtz's theory was more favored by the authorities. When Svaetichin (1956) demonstrated opponent processes in graded potentials of the carp retina, the scientific establishment was as skeptical of him as it had been of Hering. The controversial result was soon confirmed and repeated, however, and the opponent-process principle was later extended to the primate visual system in a brilliant series of electrophysiological papers by DeValois and co-workers (reviewed by DeValois and Jones, 1961), who showed that both Helmholtz and Hering had been essentially correct, the former at the receptor level and the latter at more central levels. The dispute was like that of the blind philosophers who upon encountering an elephant for the first time each felt a different part of it and then disagreed about its description, one believing it to be flexible and emitting air, another thinking it rough and columnar, etc. Though each was accurate in his own observations, it took a broader view to unite the disparate interpretations.

In his 60's, but still vigorous and productive, Hering returned to a chair at Leipzig and completed his scientific career while retaining the rigorous approaches and attitudes revealed in this book. He remained active until his death in 1918 at the age of 84, and his final work, *Grundzüge der Lehre vom Lichtsinn (Outlines of a Theory of Light Sense),* finally appeared posthumously in 1920.

The Theory of Binocular Vision belies Boring's (1950) assertion that Hering was more a phenomenologist than a careful experimenter; much of the current book shows evidence of Hering's experimental prowess. The many cases in which Hering had the courage to disagree with most of his contemporaries, where we now know that he was essentially correct and his opposition in error, show that he was ahead of his time not only in his theories but also in the care with which he executed experiments and in the confidence which he placed in their results. Perhaps Boring was blinded by the brilliance of Hering's phenomenological descriptions, such as the lucid account here of eye movements in infants (Ch. 6).

While many of his ideas were disputed or rejected during his lifetime, Hering's influence is strongly though indirectly felt today. His feeling for the inborn behavioral and perceptual organizations which parallel inborn anatomical organizations became one of the bases of the Gestalt psychology which arose in Germany nearly a half-century after the publication of this book. The description here of the tendency to see slightly irregular figures as regular (Ch. 16), for instance, anticipates the Gestalt laws of perceptual organization. The Gestalt movement in turn provided crucial starting points for contemporary cognitive psychology. Though the Gestalt movement began during Hering's lifetime, he was too old to participate in it directly and continued to be concerned with the problems which had occupied him during the 19th century.

Another component of Hering's intellectual legacy has been kept alive by his many students and their successors, fitting into the mainstream of psychology and physiology without being specifically identified with him. In the same year that *The Theory of Binocular Vision* appeared Hering was collaborating with a young student, Breuer, in work on respiration which resulted in the discovery of the Hering-Breuer reflex (Hering, 1868b). Along with the current book it was another contribution to still-gestating control theory, for it was the first satisfactory demonstration of biological negative feedback in the modern sense (see Ullman, 1970). Breuer later became associated with another famous Vienna physician and neurologist, Sigmund Freud. Hering contributed further to psychology through his student, Franz Hillebrand, and to physiology through his son H.E. Hering's collaboration with Sherrington at the time when the latter was laying the basis for modern neurophysiology (H.E. Herring and Sherrington, 1897).

In many of his ideas and attitudes Hering seems to belong more to our own age than to his, and Hurvich (1969) has listed three ways in which a thoughtful reexamination of Hering's work could be valuable: "(a) His writings, if assimilated, could help reduce confusion and unnecessary repetition of research, even today; (b) The effort to determine why some of his findings and views were unwelcome brings one face-to-face with the fascinating problem of resistance to scientific advance by scientists themselves; and finally (c) One may find that some of his opinions and views are still ahead of the time and may pose challenging questions to researchers, even today." It is my hope that this volume will contribute to a further reevaluation of Hering's careful combination of introspection with experimentation, and of specific detail with broad principle. Such a progression would have been satisfactory to Hering, who had no illusions about personal fame or recognition: "Fruitful theories will their immortal parts to their children, while their mortal shells fall away" (1880). He ended his famous lecture on memory (1870) with the insight that "The conscious memory of man ceases with death, but the unconscious memory of nature is true and inextinguishable, and he who succeeds in explaining the traces of its workings will be remembered forever."

I would like to thank Dr. Leo Hurvich for generously providing the photograph for the frontispiece, Drs. Ken Nakayama and A. Terry Bahill for thorough critical readings of the translation, and Gerald Westheimer for illuminating conversations. The work could not have been completed without efforts beyond the call of duty by Cynthia Cowee, Polly McKeever and Pat Patterson. Finally I am indebted to Diane Bridgeman, to Ewald Hering, and to my editor, Seymour

Weingarten, whose combination of enthusiasm and patience has greatly facilitated the completion of the book.

My coeditor, Lawrence Stark, wishes to dedicate this translation to the School of Optometry at the University of California, Berkeley.

Bruce Bridgeman
Santa Cruz, California
March 1976

Translator's Note

The subtlety of Hering's thought is revealed as much in his grammatical style as in his scientific reasoning. This creates a challenge for translators, for the German language has rich possibilities for subtleties which can be translated poorly or not at all into English, and Hering seemed to take advantage of all of them. (Helmholtz, in contrast, had a clear and direct style which lends itself easily to English translation; the perpetual opponents, Helmholtz and Hering, contrast even in this arena.) The current translation required extensive rearranging and simplifying of Hering's style, and many compromises had to be made. My bias was to try to err on the side of clarity of presentation at the expense of literalness of translation; the English version has considerably more and shorter sentences than the original. Most of the problems which deserve comment, however, deal with translations of specific words.

Because the vocabulary of physiological optics was just developing in Hering's time, the German text contains some inconsistencies and ambiguities in terminology. I have attempted to resolve these by using the modern equivalent English terms. One important example of this concerns the notation for rotations of the eye about the line of sight as an axis, which are translated here as cyclorotations. Hering devoted several notes to defining the German terminology for cyclorotation, naming it rolling (Rollung) to avoid the ambiguities of Helmholtz's term circular rotation (Raddrehung). The current state of cyclorotation is called the cyclorotary position here; Hering usually referred to it as orientation (Orientirung). Hering's original terms are sometimes translated literally where they do not introduce ambiguity.

There is another new word, "bifixation," which best describes the fixation of the double eye. Though Hering did not have such a word, it often seems to best describe his intent and it adds to the clarity of many sections.

In the translation of some terms I have attempted to retain the feeling which a mid-nineteenth-century German reader would have had. "Vertical dividing lines" is a literal translation of "Vertikale Trennungslinien," the lines which vertically bisect the retina while lying in a plane which contains the line of sight. Carl A. Radde has used both "vertical dividing lines" and "vertical mid-sections" for this in his 1942 translation of Hering's *Spatial Sense*. Recreating the original feeling was sometimes impossible, however; "double eye" is one word ("Doppelauge") in German, and the unitary nature of this concept is difficult to bring out in the highly analytical English syntax.

For many technical terms I have followed J.P.C. Southall's usage in his authoritative translation of Helmholtz's *Physiological Optics.* One which deserves a comment is "Drehstreben," literally "rotation striving" or "attempted rotation," which Southall has translated as "rotational force."

Often Hering used several redundant systems of terminology, a practice which I have attempted to minimize in translating. In naming the eye muscles he used three separate systems of notation, two Latin and one German, which are simplified to the standard modern usage. The four rectus muscles are "lateral rectus," "medial rectus," "superior rectus," and "inferior rectus," while the two obliques are "superior oblique" and "inferior oblique."

The references, which originally appeared as footnotes at the bottom of each page, have been grouped together at the end of the text. They appear just as Hering gave them, with a few minor additions to improve consistency. References to Helmholtz's *Physiological Optics* which appear in the body of the text are to Southall's 1925 translation (Dover edition, 1962), while those in the reference list are to the original 1867 edition which Hering used. A few typographical errors have also been corrected.

On the Movements of the Double Eye

1. *Introduction*

Three primary relationships define the movements of the eye: the direction of the lines of sight on the current objects of attention, the cyclorotary position which the retinas assume, and the regulation of light entry and focus by internal movements of the eye.

The fixation of the lines of sight on one point brings the retinal image of that point to the place of sharpest vision, that is to the point of sight (fovea) of the retina in both eyes. With the same position of one line of sight, however, many positions are possible for the other eye and especially for its retina. If one thinks of the eye as rotated about a stationary line of sight as the axis (cyclorotation), it can assume all possible positions given one direction of the line of sight. Therefore it is necessary to know the position and movement of the retina as well as the position and movement of the lines of sight. This has also been called the *orientation* of the retina (cyclorotary position). Finally, changes in the lens and the iris *accommodate* the eye for the present distance of the objects of sight and for the amount of light entering the eye from visual space.

Insofar as investigations of focus, cyclorotary orientation, and accommodation can be accomplished in the single eye, they do not belong in the plan of this book, which is principally concerned with the relationships of the two eyes and their movements. It will not always be possible to hold strictly to this plan, for we must discuss several problems which can be solved without considering normal binocular vision. It will be clear, however, that in many ways the positions and movements of the single eye cannot be made understandable without also taking note of its relationships to the other eye. The two eyes should not ordinarily be seen as two separate organs steered by the same commands, but so to say as two halves of a *single* organ. Its internal construction naturally cannot be conceived in the formerly customary gross anatomical way.

2. *On the Equal Innervation of Both Eyes*

The two eyes are so related to one another that one cannot be moved independently of the other; rather, the musculature of both eyes reacts simultaneously to one and the same impulse of will. Therefore we are usually unable to raise or lower one eye without the other. Both eyes are raised and lowered simultaneously and with equal strength. We are just as unable to innervate the muscles of one eye alone for the purpose of right or left movement, though it is possible for us to move both eyes simultaneously about different angles and with different speeds to the left or right, to move inward or outward, and even to move one eye outward or inward while the other remains still. We are able to do this not because we simultaneously give each eye a special innervation, but because in these movements each eye receives two different innervations. One is a turning of *both* eyes to the right or left and the other is inward or outward turning of *both* eyes. Since these two innervations of the double eye (Doppelauge) work together in one eye and oppositely in the other, the resultant movement in each eye must necessarily be different.

For instance, if both eyes (Fig. 1) look straight ahead for a great distance, and an object *a* at the right and very near attracts our attention, we must first direct the double eye to the proper distance and there occurs an innervation of both eyes for convergence. Through this innervation, which pulls both eyes equally strongly inward, the originally parallel lines of sight λl and ρr are directed to the points *a* and *a* at approximately equal distances, as the dashed lines $\lambda l'$ and $\rho r'$ indicate. In addition, because the object which we want to see clearly appears at the right, we must move the double eye to the right. For this an innervation of both eyes occurs for turning to the right, through which (because it affects both eyes equally) both eyes are turned to the right by the same angle, and the lines of sight finally come to the dotted lines $\lambda l''$ and pr''. Now both innervations occur simultaneously, and therefore the left line of sight receives first a command for turning inward through the angle $l\lambda l'$ and second a command for turning right through the angle $l\lambda l''$. As a result of this double command, the left line of sight is rotated to the right through $\measuredangle l\lambda l' + \measuredangle l\lambda l'' = \measuredangle l\lambda l'''$ and is therefore directed toward point *a.* The right line of sight receives first a command for inward turning through $\measuredangle r\rho r'$ and second a command for right turning through $\measuredangle r\rho r''$, both commands working in opposite directions. Because the line of sight moves in the direction of the stronger command to the right and specifically through $\measuredangle r\rho r'' - \measuredangle r\rho r' = \measuredangle r\rho r'''$ it will be positioned at point *a.* So in spite of the equally strong innervations on both eyes, a different movement of each eye results because the

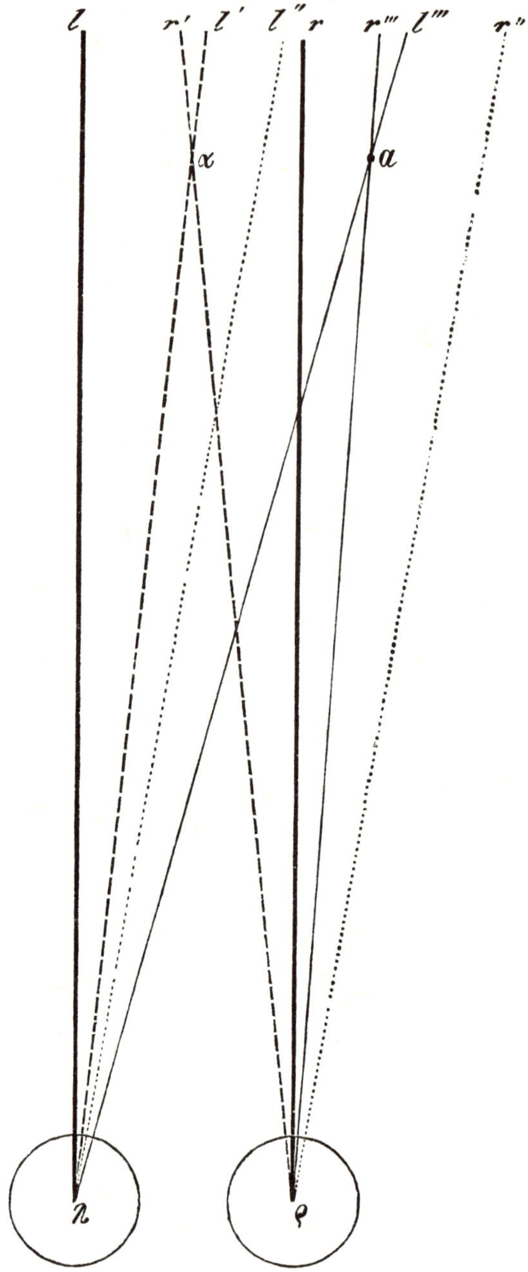

Fig. 1.

two innervations reinforce one another in one eye and inhibit each other in the other. The proofs for the accuracy of this statement will be given in the following paragraphs.

As far as their movements in the service of the sense of sight are concerned, both eyes will be handled as a single organ. To the mobilizing will it is irrelevant that this organ really consists of two separate parts because it is not necessary to move each part separately; rather, one and the same impulse of will directs both eyes simultaneously as one can direct a pair of horses with single reins.

This double eye, set into motion through single impulses of will, can be aimed at any point p in visual space so that the two lines of sight intersect at this point. The point therefore is imaged on the *points of sight of the retinas.* The point p becomes the *fixation point of the double eye* because fixation is directed to it and rests there. This bifixation is made easier from the beginning because both lines of sight lie in one plane, the *visual plane of the double eye.* Since both eyes usually rise and sink together they remain in one plane. For purely mechanical reasons, to be explained later, only with strongly raised or lowered and simultaneously sidewards directed vision do the two lines of sight not remain in one plane if the head is forcibly held steady. With usual vision this is not the case because the head and the whole body assist the movements of the double eye and make it possible that the lines of sight can always intersect.

We want to illustrate the direction which the point of sight assumes in relation to our head, that is, the visual direction of the double eye, which joins the point of sight with a point mid-way between the two eyes. This line will be called the *fixation line of the double eye* or the *binocular fixation line.* It changes position whenever our gaze wanders to the right or left or above or below, but gaze can also move along the stationary fixation line to greater nearness or greater distance.

From now on we can think of both eyes as a single imaginary eye which lies midway between the two real eyes. If such an eye had to be innervated to turn to the left, right, above or below, the two real eyes would always be equally innervated, and if such an eye had to be innervated to accommodate for greater nearness or distance, both eyes would be innervated not only for an internal accommodation but also for an external bifixation of both lines of sight for nearness or distance.

Let the fixation point lie at a (Fig. 2) and let m be the fixation of the imaginary eye accommodated for the nearness of point a, whose convergence angle $\lambda a \rho$ expresses the lines of sight of the real eyes. Now an object at b to the right and further away than a attracts the attention. In order to see it clearly, it would be necessary for the

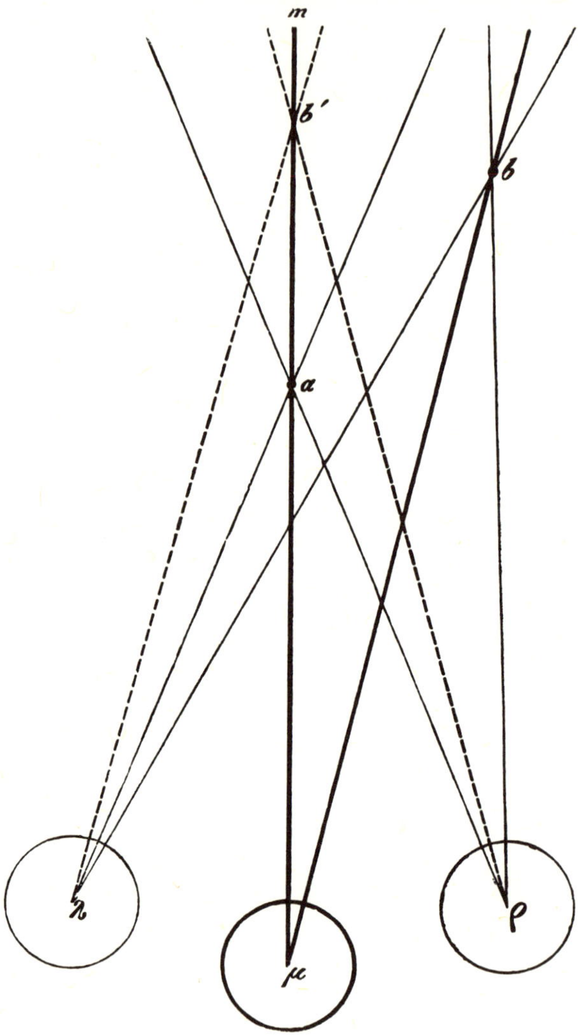

Fig. 2.

imaginary eye first to accommodate for greater distance and second to turn to the right about the angle $m\mu b$. Through accommodation alone the imaginary eye would be accommodated for the point b'. This accommodation of the imaginary eye involves in reality the accommodation of *both* eyes and at the same time the focusing of both lines of sight on the point b'. Turning the fixation line of the imaginary eye through the angle $m\mu b$ involves in the real eyes a turning of both lines of sight through an equal angle. The lines of sight, already thought of as being focused on b', must therefore rotate through the angles $b'\lambda b$ and $b'\rho b$ respectively, which are equal to $m\mu b$. As in the imaginary eye, the accommodation and the rightward turning occur not after one another but with one another; the analogous changes occur in the real double eye simultaneously. The left eye thereby receives first a command to the left corresponding to innervation of the double eye for reducing the convergence angle, and second a stronger command to the right corresponding to the innervation of the double eye for the purpose of turning right. Its line of sight therefore moved in the direction of the stronger command through the angle $b'\lambda b$ - $a\lambda b' = a\lambda b$ to the right. The right eye receives the analogous commands which, however, add to one another so that it is turned about the angle $a\rho b' + b'\rho b = a\rho b$.

In a later section the facts which are briefly sketched here will be discussed further and their meaning for spatial perception will be especially investigated. Many other supporting facts will come to light in addition to those given in the following paragraphs.

It will further be argued that the localization of the retinal images of both eyes, to the degree that they are dependent on the position and movement of the eyes at all, are not oriented for specific positions of both eyes but for the position and motion of the fixation line of the double eye, and that we not only innervate both eyes as we would innervate the single imaginary eye but that we also localize the direction of retinal images as though both real retinal images lay on the retina of the imaginary eye. This will indicate the previously unrecognized general harmony between the sensory and motor functions of the eyes, without whose understanding a satisfactory symptomology of motility disturbances is unthinkable.

Long ago simple observation had led to the general thesis that the musculature of one eye could be voluntarily innervated without the simultaneous innervation of the musculature of the other. The linking of various eye muscles for common efforts was proposed as a direct example of the so-called coordinations (Mitbewegungen); "the importance of coordinations," said Johannes Müller (24), "is that voluntary intention on one nerve calls forth involuntary intention on another. The appearances of the coordinations are not practiced, they are inborn. This coordination is the greatest among the unpracticed, and the purpose of practice and education of muscle movements is to learn to isolate single groups of fibers. The result of practice in the light of coordination is a suspension of the tendency to coordinations. It is quite different with the associations of voluntary movements. Here through practice muscles are educated for quick succession or simultaneity of movement. The result of practice with the association of movements is exactly the reverse of that with coordinations. Through practice muscles lose their inborn tendency to coordination: through practice voluntary coordination is made easier." With these words Müller distinguishes the two kinds of coordination, the involuntary, inborn movement and the voluntary, practiced association of movements. Müller took the coordination of the eyes to be inborn, and this opinion had universal acceptance until recent times when a number of opthalmologists, headed at present by Helmholtz, assigned to each eye initial complete independence from the movement of the other. This new, and as will be shown, false view developed from the opposition begun by Wheatstone against the theory of the identity of the retinas, and was a necessary consequence of the old hypothesis already proposed in substance by Descartes, and recently defended by Porterfield, Schopenhauer, Wundt, Nagel and others. According to this view we see external objects singly in spite of doubled retinal images because we project the images outward along their direction lines (or visual lines, retina normals) to their intersections.

In *Beiträge zur Physiologie* No. 123, p. 316, I have described the important law of the equal innervation of both eyes in spite of unequal movement or asymmetrical convergence as discussed above. This rule is of fundamental importance for the understanding of eye movements.

3. *Grounds For and Against the Assumption of an Always Equal Innervation of Both Eyes*

The observation that both eyes usually move together is not an adequate reason for the assumption that there is some kind of compulsion (Zwang) to simultaneous movement. The fact can be adequately explained because we must always fixate both eyes on the subject in order to see as clearly as possible and grasp the object of sight with both eyes just as we grasp and hold fast to some objects with both hands. One comes to the assumption of a compulsory link of the eyes for common movement much more through the experience that this linking also occurs when vision is not helped by it and even when it is decidedly hindered. These circumstances are principally the following:

1. If we cover one eye, the covered eye follows the movements of the other, as one can easily convince oneself by observing the loosely covered eye of a second person from the side. The will does not inhibit these coordinations, which are useless for seeing.

2. When one eye is completely blinded, it nonetheless accompanies the movements of the still-seeing one. When both eyes are fully blinded, they still always move together.

3. Squinters, who demonstrably perceive only the image of one eye, still move both eyes together.

4. The involuntary movements of nystagmus occur in both eyes simultaneously and in analogous fashion.

5. With paralysis of certain eye muscles the patients, although extremely annoyed by double images, are not able to focus the eyes on specific points, even when they are able to focus each eye singly on those points. If they could move each eye independently of the other it would be possible to simultaneously focus both eyes on all of the points on which they could focus each eye singly.

These adequately determined facts prove that coordinations also occur when they do not aid vision or even interfere with it. It follows that there is a certain *compulsion* to these coordinations.

On the other side, however, there are also facts which at first glance do not seem consistent with the asumption of such a compulsion and therefore have been used to oppose it.

If it is indeed correct that both eyes are always innervated together, it would be most likely from the beginning that the related muscles of both eyes are also always equally strongly innervated, or that at least it does not lie within our power to determine the amount of innervation for each eye separately. Otherwise it would be difficult to see why we could not reduce the innervation of one eye nearly to nothing while the amount of innervation of the other eye had any desired value. In that case the actual movements of one eye would be practically independent from those of the other. Now one would think that the compulsion for always equal innervation of both eyes would make it impossible for us to move both eyes simultaneously about different angles and with different speeds, or even to just move one eye while the other stands still. To the degree that only movements to the right and left, that is so-called lateral movements are concerned, the above facts can be brought into agreement with the assumption of always equal innervation of both eyes as explained in chapter one. But it remains to be proved that the representation given there is the only correct one, and this all the more, as it has been determined and can be introduced against my conception that we are also in a position to raise and lower one eye slightly while the other stands unmoved. Finally, the assumption of an always equal innervation of both eyes cannot be agreed upon in the same way as in the case of the inequality of the movements of both eyes to the right or left because in this case, unlike that one, we cannot assume a competition of two different innervations of the double eye.

4. *Proofs for Equal Innervation with Unequal Lateral Movement*

In Chapter 2 it was shown how the simultaneous but unequal lateral movements of both eyes or the lateral movement of only one eye while the other stood still could be easily reconciled with the assumption of an always equal innervation of both eyes. A markedly unequal lateral movement occurs only when the new fixation point appears not simply sideways from the originally fixated point but also nearer or further away so that it requires bringing the point of vision nearer or further as well as sidewards turning. If we now wanted to explain such an unequal lateral movement of both eyes from the ability to innervate both eyes simultaneously by different amounts, we would come into contradiction with the experiences recounted above which irrefutably support the assumption of a compulsion to both eyes always being innervated together. A group of direct proofs can be added to this indirect proof for the correctness of my assumption, which I will illustrate with a special example.

At the start, the double eye will be focused on a very distant point lying straight ahead so that the lines of sight (λl and ρr, Fig. 3) lie parallel. Now fixation is moved to a nearer point p to the left of the median plane and on the line of sight of the left eye. Here by my assumption first an innervation of both eyes is necessary to increase the convergence angle; if executed alone this innervation would focus the lines of sight on the locations $\rho r'$ and $\lambda l'$ and on the point p' at about the same distance as p. At the same time, however, a leftward turning of the double eye is necessary to bring the binocular line of sight μm from its middle position to the position $\mu m'$. This is an innervation which if it occurred alone would move both lines of sight to the left through an angle equal to the angle $m\mu m'$ so that they would come to the positions $\rho r'$ and $\lambda l''$. Both innervations take place simultaneously, so that the left eye receives simultaneously two equally strong impulses working directly against one another and consequently yields neither to one nor to the other but remains in position. In the right eye the two equal impulses for movement work in the same direction, so that this eye is pulled twice as far to the left as each of the two innervations would move it singly, and its line of sight comes to the corresponding position r'''. Both lines of sight are now focused on the point p. Thus, assuming the appropriate position of the fixation plane, only the adductor (medial rectus) acts on the right eye. But on the left eye the adductor is in operation as well as the abductor (lateral rectus). The left eye, because two antagonistically working muscles are operating on it, will therefore behave differently than before when its line of sight indeed had the same position but the innervation of the two mentioned antagonists was not taking

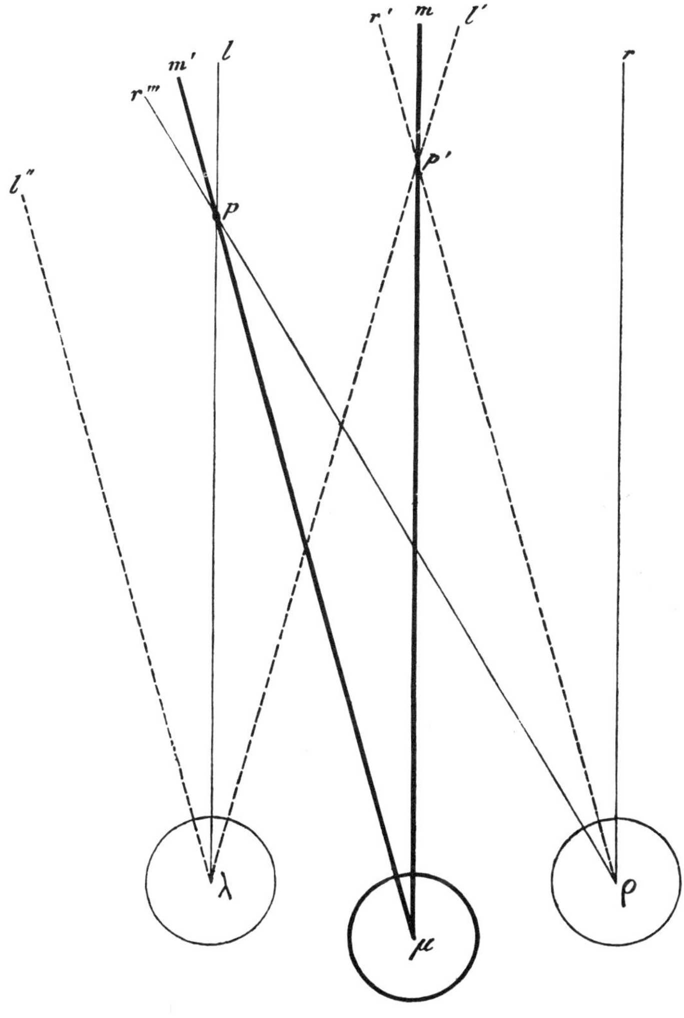

Fig. 3

place; it will be in a condition of increased tension and the intraocular pressure will increase, although the position of the line of sight remains completely the same.

A slight back and forth twitching of the left eye, which a second observer can easily perceive, reveals two antagonistic muscle forces operating in the movement described above. This twitch becomes weaker after a while if one frequently practices analogous experiments. The two concurrent innervations on the left eye understandably do not rise so mathematically exactly during the entire course of the fixation movement that a transitory short dominance of one muscle over the other cannot occur. The twitch proves that the innervation is not restricted to the right eye, but also affects the left eye, although it is already focused on the point *p* and its movement is therefore completely counterproductive.

The described unsymmetrical bifixation of the double eye on point *p* uses muscle forces other than those in effect when the left eye is fixated on a very distant point with the same position of the left line of sight. The left eye might also have a slightly different total position. Its retina especially might be differently located, in spite of the equal position of its line of sight in both cases. Specifically, if the pulling forces of the adductor on one side and of the abductor on the other are not diametrically opposed, a small moment of rotation must result from these two forces in a manner to be described later, and the line of sight would be slightly deviated from its position if a compensation from other muscle actions did not intervene. In short, in one case the line of sight would be maintained by muscle forces other than those present in the other case. Such a difference in the active pulling forces on the eye could, however, lead to a different position of the retina, that is, the orientation of the eye. Experiments can prove that a difference in orientation actually occurs in both cases, though the above-noted simultaneous tension of the lateral and medial recti is by no means the only cause of this difference. We will see later that the rule of orientation for the double eye focused on a distant point is different than for focus on near objects.

Because the right line of sight moves to the left in the case just discussed, while the left does not move except for small twitches, there is a small cyclorotation of the left eye. This proves that the left eye is held in its final position by different muscle activities and therefore by a different innervation than before, although the position of its line of sight did not change.

With near vision, by my assumption, as soon as the point of sight no longer lies in the medial plane, one eye must always be under the influence of antagonistic innervation. Specifically, this is the eye on the side to which the point of sight deviates from the median

plane. First the adductor of this eye will be innervated corresponding to the nearness of the point of sight, and second the abductor will be innervated corresponding to the *sideward deviation* of the point of sight from the median plane. Thus if we hold a piece of paper parallel to the facial plane and close to the face, and let our vision wander back and forth on it, both adductors will be continuously innervated, and each time the point of vision leaves the median plane to the right or left, the abductor of the right or left eye respectively is also innervated. If one tries, for instance, to look as far to the left as possible under these conditions, the abductor of the left eye is not able to turn the eye as far to the left as it is with distant vision, where the adductor of the same eye is not innervated. It is therefore under less tension and opposes the abductor with less resistance. This result of our assumption agrees with experience: *the maximum excursion of the left eye to the left and the right eye to the right is smaller with near vision than with far vision.* The nearer the field of vision lies to the eye the smaller it becomes. This fact would be unexplainable if each eye were innervated independently.

To demonstrate the reduction of the field with near accommodation in the left eye, for instance, one can produce a lasting afterimage of a small disk or of a fixated small vertical strip of colored paper on the place of direct vision. Now one goes to a window with a free view and steadies his head position by biting on a small well-anchored board mounted horizontally; one then turns the left eye to the left, pays attention to the afterimage and notes the distant object O to which one can move it. On the windowpane, which must be very near the eye, one marks the point P where the line of sight to the object O in question intersects the window. If one now accommodates the eyes for the near window pane, on which one has made small points or lines as fixation objects, one is no longer able to move the afterimage to the point P at the left. This is again possible, however, when one accommodates for distance. The latter control is necessary because the excursion ability of the eye declines very quickly from fatigue, and one obtains false results if one does not switch the accommodations from nearness to distance several times successively. It is not advisable to perform this experiment without an afterimage because only the afterimage gives us certain information about the present position of the line of sight. Without an afterimage one usually over-estimates the excursion ability and therefore holds an indirectly seen object to be still directly seen, because it is the sole object of our attention at the time.

If we direct only one eye, for instance the left, to a very distant point lying directly in front of us, and then bring a pinpoint P into the line of sight a few inches away from the eye and attempt to see it

clearly, the line of sight of the left eye does not have to change its position but only its state of refraction. The double eye here behaves exactly as it does in the example of Fig. 3. First, the covered right eye is positioned to the pinpoint and second, the left eye makes the same twitches which we learned about above. By our hypothesis, this is quite understandable; one case, like the other, concerns transferring of vision from a very far point lying straight ahead to a nearer one lying to the left. For this purpose the double eye is innervated in the same way in both cases. It is irrelevant for the innervation that in one case the right eye does not participate in the act of seeing, for this innervation is not isolated to one eye or the other.

I have already mentioned that the direction in which a fixated object appears ordinarily corresponds to the current position of the line of sight of the double eye. In the experiment described here, the line of sight of the double eye changes position in that innervation directed to the double eye is turned to the left. As a result, the pinpoint correspondingly appears to the left of the median plane although the line of sight of the left eye (the only one seeing) has not changed its position at all. It therefore seems that as long as both lines of sight lie parallel, both the fixated distant object and the pinpoint covered with its blur circles lie directly before us in the median plane, but as soon as we have accommodated the left eye for the pinpoint both objects seem to lie to the left, corresponding to the changed position of the line of sight of the double eye. During the accommodation itself, both objects undergo an apparent motion to the left. This experiment succeeds especially well if arranged in the manner described below for everyone who normally is not accustomed to the monocular use of one or the other eye. It does not have such great success if it is set up with an eye which is very frequently used monocularly. A significant condition of the experiment is that one must somehow anchor the pin so that it does not muddy the result through unsteadiness, and that one must look through a tube so as not to be disturbed by illusions about the true position of objects.

This experiment would apparently have a very different result if each eye had its own motility, because then the retinal image of each eye would have to be localized according to its own position, as many have mistakenly assumed. In that case neither the movement of the covered eye during the experiments nor the influence of its position on the localization of the image in the other eye is explainable.

These proofs for the occurrence of an always equal innervation in both eyes, in spite of unequal movement or asymmetrical convergence, will be adequate for the present. It is anticipated that the observations and experiments described here may vary in many ways.

One can arrange the experiment described above in the following way. Two parallel tubes, 6-8 inches long and 1 inch wide, blackened on the inside, are mounted before the eyes so that the axis of each line of sight lies on the axis of one tube with the eyes directed straight ahead. On the end opposite the eye, each tube is closed by a cover which can be opened upward. The cover must close so tightly that no light can shine through. At a distance slightly exceeding the near point of the eye, a stick is inserted in each tube so far that its tip lies in the axis of the tube. The stick must be broad enough that it can still be seen as a shadow in spite of the large blur circles of its retinal image when one looks through the tube at a distant object. If one looks through these double tubes in the distance, the two visible tube openings fuse to a single one and the two sticks also appear as only one, if the tubes are at the correct distance from one another. One now fixates a distant object so that it lies directly behind the indistinctly visible stick and lets a helper apply the cover to one of the two tubes. One can now see with only one eye; now one turns his attention from the far object to the near stick and tries to see it clearly. While one does this, both the tube opening and the stick apparently move to the side and both finally appear on the right or left side, though as long as one had looked in the distance they had appeared to lie in the median plane.

As already mentioned, the experiment is not so striking if it is performed with an eye which is very frequently used monoptically, for instance in microscopy. Nonetheless, the success described also occurs in such an eye, though less clearly, and if one then uses the other eye, the success is all the more surprising. The reason for these phenomena, which are already in the realm of the abnormal, will be discussed later.

In performing the above experiment I note that as soon as I strongly accommodate, the fixated object not only makes an apparent motion in the horizontal direction outward but that it simultaneously moves downward somewhat, and finally that a fixated cross of threads also rotates slightly about its middle point such that its upper portion tips to the side of the closed eye. According to the rules which the spatial arrangement of retinal images follow, this observation must lead to the conjecture that the open eye, in accommodating for nearness, makes not only an involuntary movement inward but also suffers a weaker one upward. As already noted, the first movement is neutralized through a voluntary innervation of the lateral rectus. In order to correct the latter also, the muscles which lower the eye must also be innervated. Finally, the innervation necessary to maintain the visual direction at the height of the fixation point results in the apparent movement downward.

The apparent cyclorotation of the line of sight suggests the conjecture that the observing eye experiences a small cyclorotation during accommodation for nearness, specifically in the direction opposite to the rotation of the field of vision. This accommodation-induced cyclorotation will be thoroughly discussed later.

5. *On the Artificial Upward or Downward Deviation of One Eye*

I have referred above to one more fact which appears to speak against the hypothesis of always equal innervation of both eyes. If we hold a very weak prism with the base up or down in front of one eye, a previously fixated point appears in double images lying over one another, though they flow together after a while. The double images fuse because the eye behind the prism is rotated slightly upward or downward, so that both lines of sight no longer lie in one plane. It is best to arrange the experiment so that the weak prism is first held with the base outward and then, after simple vision is re-achieved, is slowly rotated about the line of sight until the base lies exactly upward or downward (Donders). The more often one performs this experiment, the stronger the prism which one can use in this way. I have myself used a prism mounted in an eye-glass frame and have gone to continuously stronger prisms and finally compensated for one of eight degrees, though only with great effort and for a very short time.

This observation that one can turn one line of sight slightly upward or downward, while the other remains in position, can also be made in stereoscopic experiments if the occasion arises. It is known that one can fuse two stereoscopic images without any apparatus if one places the lines of sight parallel so that they meet corresponding points on both images. If one is near-sighted and brings both images to the range of the far point of the eyes, one sees the fused image in optimal focus. If one now rotates the paper with the two images while observing the fused image, and holds the head steady so that one image comes to lie higher than the other, or if one turns the head slightly about a forward-backward axis without moving the images, the fusion of both images is still possible to a certain degree because one line of sight goes slightly upward and the other slightly downward. Or if one cuts the paper with the images into two halves and pushes one image slowly upward or downward while the head is fixed, the images can similarly remain fused up to a certain threshold of misalignment. Here also one observes that long practice allows a fused image with a larger difference in heights.

These experiments do not concern fused vision with non-corresponding retinal locations. Rather, the different heights of the lines of sight actually permit fused vision. It follows that when one suddenly removes the prism or the stereoscopic images after a while, the objects behind them appear doubled at first because the lines of sight come back only gradually to the same plane, as one can recognize clearly when the vertically displaced double images approach one another. The longer the experiment has lasted, the more slowly the lines of sight return to their normal positions. After a very short-duration observation, and if the deviation was small, it usually occurs so fast that it can easily escape observation.

These facts cannot be brought into agreement with the assumption of always equal innervation of both eyes in the same way as those in the previous paragraphs; however, they cannot prove that this compulsion does not exist, but only illustrate that the compulsion is not entirely irresistible. If we observe other coordinations, we will find that they behave in an analogous manner throughout. Everywhere there is a more or less important tendency for several muscles to act together. This tendency is sometimes so strong that it appears to us as an irresistible compulsion. After long, tiring, and fruitless experiments, we finally succeed for a while in finding the innervation through which the operation of one muscle can be made slightly independent from another. I needed much practice before I succeeded in closing one eye independently of the other, and today, in spite of years of practice, I am still not able to close one without a twitch of the lid of the other (which I did not notice at all until I once performed the experiment before a mirror). This one example illustrates many others. Who after this could assert, for instance, that each eyelid has an innervation fully independent of that of the other? In the same way, the experiments just mentioned cannot prove anything about the motor independence of both eyes; rather, they themselves show clearly that the tendency to raise or lower both eyes together is very great and can be overcome only slightly and with great effort, so that one can truly speak of a compulsion. If one were unwilling to admit the existence of coordinations as such because it is possible through fortune or practice to separate one movement more or less from the others, one would be forced to dismiss a whole area of well-known facts.

Our capacity to raise or lower one eye for several degrees independently of the other contradicts the assumption that both eyes are usually equally innervated. But it does not prove anything decisively, for an absolute inviolability of this compulsion to equal innervation was not plausible from the beginning; and just because the vast majority of the coordinations known to us can be made more or less independent through practice, no one would maintain that the coordinations of the eye will be an exception to this.

That the compulsion to equal innervation can be somewhat overcome has several advantages for binocular vision, especially under abnormal conditions, as we will see later. Here again the organism shows us a mechanism which, though created with principles that are unchangeable, nonetheless has a certain ability to accommodate for changed relationships.

The seemingly automatic focusing of the lines of sight on an object which catches our attention has often been pointed out as a reflex movement; and one might think that the deviation of one line of sight in the discussed experiments occurred because the object imaged eccentrically in one eye caused a reflex deviation which would have nothing to do with the compulsion to always equal *voluntary* innervation of the eyes. Here it should first be noted that the retinal images can direct eye movements only when they are attended to and are objects of attention; thus, with unthinking vision, in spite of numerous double images, the eyes do not focus on the objects lying before us at all, while the true reflex motions are just so characterized that they occur most easily and powerfully when consciousness and attention are shut out. In any case, attention and with it the phenomenon of consciousness could make the retinal image into a reflex stimulus, and this would give us a very strange kind of reflex motion. In addition, the circumstance that the deviation of one eye can be made easier through practice does not speak for the conception of such movements as reflex movement either.

Thus when I suddenly hold a prism of, for instance, six degrees before the eye with its base up or down, I cannot compensate for it. But if I first hold the base inward or outward and slowly turn the base into the horizontal orientation I can successfully compensate the prism. Indeed, the slowness with which an eye corrects itself after deviation in the above manner is of interest. For instance, if one has held the prism before the eye for a long time one sees double images over one another for several minutes after removal of the prism, accompanied by a feeling of tension in the deviated eye. Only after weak and short-lasting deviation does the eye move quickly back into its normal position.

Helmholtz has made the following observation in his discussion of eye movement: "I have observed that when I become sleepy in the evening at reading, and double images of the lines begin to appear, these double images often stand over one another and sometimes show a rotation against one another. Thus in this condition, where the will loses its energy, and one would expect the most unhindered expression of movement tendencies prescribed by the anatomical mechanism, the usual orderliness of the eye movements ceases."

This conclusion, though it comes from an observation which is correct in itself, is inadmissible. If one becomes sleepy at reading, the eyes frequently focus on a point which is further than the paper, that is, they begin to move from a position requiring effort back into a more comfortable one. Thus double images of the letters and lines can appear next to one another only when the fixation plane coincidentally intersects the paper in a line parallel to the lines of print. In other cases, however, if one holds the head slightly tilted, for instance by supporting it on one arm, the double images must appear at different heights. Thus Helmholtz probably had not paid attention to head position in his observations, and therefore came to the conclusion that the eyes of a sleepy person no longer moved according to the rules of association, but moved independently from one another.

In his *Physiological Optics* (Vol. III, p. 59), Helmholtz has tried to defend his position against my previous objections and has extended his discussion of these double images, saying that he has observed them not only when he became tired when reading in the evening but also when he tried to hold his eyes open after a long dinner out of politeness to his company. When he roused himself, the double images quickly fused from their positions at different heights and rotated relative to one another, and when he tried again to separate them voluntarily, only the usual side-by-side double images occurred. If this is really the case and not, as is more likely, that with his arousal he straightened his head, which had nodded somewhat to the side, it proves nothing more than that Helmholtz does not have an equally fully developed muscle system in each eye, but that there is here a case of a minor motility disturbance. As one can frequently observe, this occurs only when fixation is released and the eyes are, so to say, left to themselves. Unfortunately, Helmholtz did not specify the relative positions of the double images which he observed and which apparently behave so abnormally. This information would have been all the more valuable because it concerns observations made in a state of sleepiness. With this one is not in a position to diagnose the possible motility disturbance more exactly. As is well known, people who have equally well developed muscle systems in each eye squint only laterally in a state of sleepiness, and not upward or downward. But upward or downward squinting must be assumed to explain the abnormal position of the double image given by Helmholtz. Very small differences in heights of the double images can be obtained even with an erect head if one half-closes one eye, because the bulbus is pushed slightly by the contraction of the orbicularis.

I have no objection to the idea that the eyes are under special innervation during sleep, but I do not understand why one eye should be more affected by sleepiness than the other, why, so to say, one eye should become sleepier than the other. Because no more exact information is available about this point than that which Helmholtz has given, I find no reason to give up my doubts.

6. *Proof That the Compulsion to Equal Innervation of Both Eyes Is Inborn*

It remains to investigate whether the compulsion to equal innervation of both eyes proven above is inborn or is rooted in long-standing habit. In answering this question, one must take care not to permit certain general principles for which one is prejudiced to influence the judgement. Thus, for instance, Burkhard said in his valuable work on "The sensitivity of the two eyes for double images" (2): "Whatever I can get rid of through practice and observation, I can consider as acquired by becoming accustomed to it." As I have already shown elsewhere (19), this sentence is as false as if one had said: "What I cannot get rid of through practice and careful observation, I can consider as inborn." The fact that the assumed compulsion to common innervation of both eyes cannot be overcome in any important respect does not prove that it is inborn, as already shown. For just as a man can learn bad muscle habits until they become second nature, so that he cannot suppress them again in spite of the best efforts of will, so could the usually highly practical common innervation of the eyes rest on a habit which finally cannot be given up any more in the interest of seeing, and the strong establishment of those habits would be all the more plausible because there are no muscles in the entire body, except for certain involuntary ones, which are used as frequently as the eye muscles.

On the other hand, the fact that the compulsion to common innervation can be overcome within very narrow bounds does not prove that it is learned, and Helmholtz (12) is in error when he finds in this a proof for the motor independence of the two eyes: *for most of the familiar and probably inborn coordinations show that they can be more or less overcome by the will.* Helmholtz apparently had not thought of the observations that one can make on newborn children. The newborn makes dominantly symmetrical movements, and usually raises both arms and legs together, etc.; he learns only slowly the conjugate use of symmetrical muscles which occur on both sides. From our ability to use only one of two corresponding muscles in the two halves of the body, no one would conclude that the simultaneous innervation of symmetrically placed muscles is based solely on habit and not on an inborn organization of our nervous systems. This occurs hundred of times in adults without their attention. For then analogously one would have to deny all inborn capabilities for specific combinations of movements and to trace everything back to simple practices. One would necessarily conclude that the hen in the egg and the cat in its mother's body had already learned to walk. Even though inborn coordinations are not as numerous and striking in man as in many animals, they are still numerous and constantly present. One can restrict a young four-footed animal so that it always advances both legs simultaneously like a giraffe; and when it has learned this, it walks in this way all its life. May one find here a proof that the natural gait of animals of the same type is not given from birth or made possible by inborn nervous linkages for common use, but that they have a common center or that they are excited together by the same rules of innervation?

It is therefore an incontestable experience, and I do not need to add well known examples, that inborn associations of specific nerves and muscles for common action can be more or less separated by the will; the fact that we can raise or lower one eye slightly without the other is only a further example of this, and also illustrates that some coordinations are easier to modify through the will than others.

So there is nothing which can prove the assumption of inborn coordination of the eyes even as unlikely: on the contrary, one can make many other observations which definitely prove that this is really an inborn capability.

As already mentioned, newborn children usually move symmetrical parts simultaneously. This is very clear on the face, but it is also seen in the extremities because infants pull in or reach out with both legs or both arms at the same time, twist both hands simultaneously, etc., as long as their position or other hindrances do not restrict the movement. Conversely, conjugate, and therefore unsymmetrical movements are not prominent in newborns. One notices no special tendency to move both hands simultaneously to the same side or to turn one palm up and the other down. Only the eyes are a very striking exception; they make prominent conjugate movements, and rotate together about equal angles left and right. *Thus, while symmetrical movements dominate over the entire remainder of the body, the eyes show conjugate, and therefore unsymmetrical, movements.* This forces everyone who observes it to be immediately convinced that the overall plan is so to say a symmetrical organization which is clearly seen in the movements of other body parts, but is abandoned in the very special organization of the motor system of the eyes. Further, while in newborns the extremities often differ with respect to the direction and size of their generally symmetrical movements and therefore show a certain independence in addition to the inborn tendency to coordination, *the eyes show such a precision in simultaneous raising and lowering that both lines of sight always remain in the same plane.* One should not believe that the latter is difficult to judge, because even small deviations of one eye upward are unmistakable for a practiced observer. Simple observation gives us here a measurement which, though indeed not mathematical, has fully adequate accuracy for our purpose. Finally, newborns do have some symmetrical movements, such as inward turning of both eyes, which, though indeed relatively more rare than the conjugate movements, are executed with the same exactness. I have made these observations in many newborns immediately after birth so that it is established without doubt that an inborn capability is observed.

Not every newborn child is suitable for this observation. Many have such narrow eye openings and squint constantly so much that investigation is difficult. But not infrequently there are children who lie there with wide open lids immediately after birth and display the discussed appearances most beautifully.

One could come to the supposition that the above discussed coordination of the movements of both eyes occurs because each eye has an independent reflex mechanism and that harmonious movements can be explained because one and the same object in the outer world sends its image to both eyes, therefore stimulating both retinas on approximately corresponding locations, and excites corresponding reflex movements in both eyes. This assumption has little value because newborns have no tendency at all in their eye movements to fixation of especially prominent or illuminated objects. But the assumption can be directly contradicted in that when one covers one eye with the hand held obliquely so that most external objects are invisible, but one can still see both eyes, one over and one under the hand, the same coordination of movements is present as before. This would not be possible for a one-sided reflex in each eye.

On the contrary, the latter observation gives meaning to the fact that an excitation of only one retina can excite the simultaneous reflex movement of both eyes, though this would mean only that there is an inborn linking of the motor apparatus of both eyes for common functioning. This would still have to be proved. But as mentioned, the eye movements of newborns immediately after birth do not give the impression that they are concerned with reflex-mediated fixations of objects placed before them. During the observations one comes instead to the interpretation that the impulse to movement, whatever its origin, activates both the limbs of the newborn and the eye movement. Because of the inborn linking of the motor apparatus of both eyes, they react simultaneously to the same innervation. The observation proves *that the coordination of the movements of the two eyes is based on an inborn ability and not on practice.*

This also explains the experience that even in children who are otherwise very capable of learning and show great ability for accommodation, the association of certain eye movements is so inborn that in pathological cases the act of coordinated seeing is given up. Squinting occurs instead of the dissociation of this coordination to more than a certain degree. At least it would be striking if children were already led by simple habit to so strong a compulsion that it could not be overcome even when it immediately ran against the interest of the act of seeing.

It is apparent that the always equal and simultaneous innervation of both eyes must make use of the eyes very much earlier, be it for equal movements toward only one side, or symmetrical movements, or for a mixed movement resulting from both kinds of motor impulses. Because of this, in order to use both eyes functionally the child need not seek the innervation of the other eye in order to innervate the first, and then painstakingly practice the simultaneous excitation of these two innervations in countless combinations. On the contrary, to a will bent on clear vision, the doubled eye is only one organ. It does not need a special location, excitation, and goal for each of its two halves, but is mastered through single impulses.

In order to appreciate the advantages of this arrangement, one should compare the long practice and effort which the student must spend before it is possible for him to play the piano with both hands simultaneously with precision; how effortfully in general all purely conjugate movements of the extremities are learned. Here for every innervation of one hand, the corresponding innervation for the other must be found and these countless combinations must be mastered. And now think how easy these conjugate movement of the extremities are compared to the reciprocal movements, because they are prescribed in the inborn organization of the motor system (although not nearly as decisively as in the eyes). In the child it is obvious how slowly the inborn relationships of symmetrical movements are dissociated, and how the reciprocal unsymmetrical movement of both arms and hands is first learned much later. If one gives an adult the task of moving both raised hands simultaneously right and left in quick succession, one sees what difficulties this very simple movement creates as he uses the forearms and the whole body for help. Despite these efforts he reverts quickly and involuntarily to symmetrical movements so that both hands move simultaneously inward or outward instead of together left and right. One is able to write fairly well with the left hand if one writes from right to left, especially when the other hand writes the same word simultaneously in the usual way from left to right; here the movements of both hands are symmetrical. But if one tries to write from left to right with both hands or even with the left alone one will see that this is significantly more difficult.

Corresponding with the inborn structures described here, the child also learns to grasp external objects with the eyes, hold them fast, and follow them with eye movements much sooner than he can grasp and hold anything with the hand. He fixates an object moved back and forth before his eyes with his attention strongly and surely directed to it when he is still a long way from even a rudimentary mastering of the movements of his hands. Thus, we see eye movements much earlier than the movements of the organs of touch, in slavish service of the sense of vision and as true companions of the attention directed to visual objects.

7. *On the Motives of Eye Movement*

Our eye movements are usually directed by spatial perceptions or conceptions; indirectly and thus unclearly seen objects which excite our attention, and therefore the effort to see them more clearly, are the most frequent triggers of eye movement. A *spatial* perception precedes the movement of the eyes and determines their direction. The simple conjecture of an object present somewhere which triggers eye movements is much less frequent; here a *conception* of the location where one supposes the object to be precedes the movement and determines its direction. *Striving for the clearest possible perception of an object combined with the perception or conception of its position relative to the object just observed determines our eye movement.* This does not include the eye movements which are not in the interest of vision but result from other conditions such as affect.

The will reveals itself in the area of the sense of sight as so-called attention that in this context is the effort to sharpen perception of the objects of sight. With respect to sensitivity, this effort has the result that from the great number of light impressions which grows simultaneously into consciousness, those which are closely related to objects of attention move into consciousness more easily, clearly and lastingly than the others. But the result of the movement is that the eyes assume so to say by themselves the position and focus by which the object of attention receives the greatest possible clarity. We are not aware of our eye movements in the same way that we are aware of the movements of our extremities, for instance, and only if we are made aware of the relationship between the position of the eyes and the position of the observed object in other people do we receive an indirect idea of the corresponding position of the eyes. Thus with vision our will is not organized to bring the eyes into any particular position, and a conception of the position of the eyes cannot determine the proper direction of movement.

The movements of the eyes executed in the service of the sense of sight are therefore not voluntary in the sense that the raising and lowering of an arm is under some circumstance, for here the will can really be directed to give the arm a previously conceived position, which is not the case with the eye; but they are also not involuntary in the sense that they occur without the participation of the will. The will is here much more the *causa movens.* The goal of the will is not the eye position in itself but the clear perception of an object of sight; the movement is not willed as such but it is directed by will, and is therefore voluntary.

Most people cannot converge the eyes when they have only distant objects in front of them and cannot place the eyes parallel when only near objects are visible. But they can succeed at both if they can clearly imagine in the first case a near object and in the second a distant object. We are simply accustomed to moving the eyes only in the service of spatial perception and therefore need such a perception, or at least a spatial concept, to set the eyes in motion and to direct their movements.

The inner relationship between spatial perception or conception and eye movement is shown especially well with the direction of attention to a more peripherally lying retinal image without moving the eyes. The unpracticed are almost totally unable to do this; their eyes move constantly with their attention and immediately place themselves on the object to which attention is directed. Practice is necessary to make the direction of attention more or less independent of the direction of the eyes. I am successful only if I pay attention to both the directly and indirectly seen objects together for as soon as attention is directed mostly to the indirectly seen objects the eyes begin a corresponding movement. Similarly, afterimages and *mouches volantes* (fleeting flies, "floaters" in the vitreous humor – B.B.*) are very instructive in this context. As soon as attention is directed to an afterimage or a *mouche volante* which appears not in the direction of vision but to one side, the eye immediately glides in the direction in which the apparent object lies, but without catching it, because the latter seems to slide away in the same direction as the eye follows it. The relationship between spatial conceptions and eye movement is also demonstrated in the effort for clear perception of an object which is imagined or conceived to be visible somewhere but is not at all present, being solely a general conception of a specific spatial relationship in consciousness. Individuals who possess a lively mimicry lift the eyes like the hand when they speak of spatially high or even only conceptually exalted things and accompany all spatial conceptions with correspondingly directed movements of the eyes and other limbs.

Eye movements generally concern transferring the eyes from one fixated object to another already more or less distinctly perceived one. The spatial relationship between the goal point of the movement and the currently observed object determines the type of innervation and thus the direction of movement of the binocular point of vision. *Except for the desire to displace the fixation point in general, the determiner of innervation is a more or less clear grasp of the position of the goal point of the movement relative to the present fixation point.* Here only the real or apparent relative position

*We thank Prof. R. Mandell for this literal and literary translation from the French.

of two external objects is relevant; only if the movement is directed to a real or apparent object which is not yet directly seen but is merely guessed or conceived somewhere can the relative position of the latter to our body sometimes determine the movement alone. This is seen when an odor elicits the urge to explore the nature of some object in a specific direction. Such cases are relatively infrequent and deserve no further discussion here.

The directing of eye movements concerns much less the determination of the absolute distance between the goal point of the movement and the present point of sight than it does the approximately correct grasp of the *direction* in which one lies relative to the other; for if the point of sight is simply pushed forward in the proper direction it will arrive at its goal in any case. It does not damage the accuracy of our movements that judgements about the absolute size of the distance of an indirectly seen object from the present object of fixation are inaccurate, and that a correct estimate is first possible when the point of sight has already moved on the path between the two objects. The direction of the indirectly seen object relative to the present fixated point is already grasped correctly, even before the movement, within very small error tolerances.

As will be discussed later in numerous examples we note with exact investigation that the grasp of the absolute distances of things, from one another as well as from our bodies, is very incomplete if the specifics of the visual space are not already known to us from earlier experience. This incompleteness occurs especially with the first look into a previously unknown visual space, while it disappears more and more when our vision has explored the various directions of the visual space. It follows that our exact orientation with respect to the true positions of objects in space is a result of eye movement, and that the confidence with which we move our fixation from object to object is probably not a result of our previous exact orientation with respect to their absolute positions.

Many examples in later sections will show that even our grasp of the position of a *fixated* object relative to the body is very unsure with respect to both distance and direction, if we cast our gaze in a space whose objects do not make possible a judgement of their position from earlier experience. On the contrary, we grasp the exact *positions* of single successively fixated objects relative to one another, not with respect to their absolute distances but with respect to the directions in which one lies relative to another. We perceive the relationships which the single distances have to one another even when the aid of further experiences about the objects of sight is entirely impossible.

All of this shows that in governing our eye movements and the innervations necessary for them we are dedicated preferentially to the grasp of the direction in which each object lies relative to others. This is true whether the goal of the motion is right or left of the presently fixated object, higher or lower, nearer or further, or any other relationship of possible combinations of these various directions. Conversely, a correct estimate of the absolute distance of objects from one another as well as the direction in which they lie relative to our *heads* does not aid the purposeful direction of the eyes.

Although the prospect of seeing a somewhere visible or imagined object clearly is the most frequent motive of eye movements, they can also be set into voluntary motion for completely different reasons. I myself, for instance, did not learn converging squint as a child by imagining a very close object but by a completely different method. One boy entertained other boys with his voluntary squinting. I tried to do the same as he, and after many unsuccessful tries was suddenly lucky, as I recognized from the applause that I earned. The peculiar feeling which I then had in the eyes and which eyeryone receives with excessive convergence of the lines of sight has served me ever since as a clue whenever I wanted to squint inward. I needed only to think of this feeling to strive to reproduce it, and immediately squinting occurred without my ever having had to think that a very near object was before me. Later when I had the need to place my eyes parallel in spite of a near object during optical experiments, I could not succeed by imagining a distant object. On the contrary, one evening as I became tired during reading I noted that I repeatedly received asymmetrical double images as soon as my attention to the reading material slackened. I saw then that I could voluntarily call forth these double images as soon as I gave up my effort to see the letters clearly, and since then I have always produced the reduction of the convergence of the lines of sight by so to say leaving the eyes to themselves and giving up the effort to see clearly. Of course I did not always bring the eyes to a true parallel position in this way. But when I tried to fuse double images by parallel positioning, it was easy for me to overcome the last bit of convergence because the double images approaching each other attracted the eyes so to say by themselves into parallelism, as they always do in ordinary vision, so that there are not really any abnormal conditions here. Immediately thereafter it was still impossible for me to reach the goal of parallel lines of sight when I really had only single near objects before me. Gradually, however, I learned to force the unequal double images on the two sides voluntarily further and further from one another, which cost me much effort at the beginning, but never and still not today did I ever use the conception of a very far object as an aide to reach parallelism. The idea of forcing the present double images further and further from one another was always with me when I wanted to further reduce the convergence angle of the lines of sight which I had already reduced by simply leaving the eyes to themselves.

Similarly, I did not learn monocular accommodation independent of the position of the object of sight by imagining a nearer or farther object. Excited by P.H. Weber's article on negative accommodation, I tried to see whether it was not possible for me to sharply image an object which lay somewhat beyond the true far point of my somewhat myopic eye and was thus visible only with blur circles. I did not succeed in this, but the exact opposite of my expectations occurred: my eye accommodated for greater nearness. With this I had a feeling in the eye similar to that which strong convergence of the eye causes. The memory of this feeling combined with the effort for its reproduction has made it possible for me since then to accommodate myself for nearness with monocular fixation of a different object, or to voluntarily reduce my pupil size. Conversely, I also learned to accommodate for distance during monocular observation of near objects by so to say giving up meaningful seeing and leaving the eye to itself. In like manner, I have also learned to strengthen or reduce accommodation for nearness with binocular vision without changing the convergence of the lines of sight. Here too I have never found spatial conceptions necessary for accomplishing the desired innervation.

These experiences are instructive insofar as they show the various ways in which one and the same focusing or positioning of the eyes can be voluntarily accomplished, and that it is not exclusively spatial perceptions and conceptions which call forth eye movements and determine their type even though this is the case with usual vision. They are also important in another context to be discussed later, concerning certain disharmonies between eye position and localization.

8. *On the Innervation of the Double Eye*

I define the fixation space of the double eye as the space within which the intersection of both lines of sight, that is, the binocular visual point, can be moved with unchanged head position. This fixation space is to be thought of as tightly tied to the head, and changes its position only when the head changes its position. Every point in the fixation space has, therefore, an unchangeable position relative to the head or to the points of rotation of the eyes. If each eye possessed only the four rectus muscles, it would immediately be specified which muscles and degrees of contraction would be necessary for any given position of the lines of sight in fixation space in order to hold the lines of sight, and with them the point of vision, steady in this position. Because each eye has six muscles, however, one can think of the fixation of the lines of sight in a given position as brought about in varying ways by the muscles. Fixation on one and the same point of visual space could then be maintained now with this and now with another muscle, and the various muscle actions would of course correspond to varying innervations.

In reality it does not behave this way. *Rather, the same muscles are always shortened in the same way if the point of sight again has the same position in fixation space, and fixation is always held in this position with the same innervation.* Thus in order to maintain fixation on a given point in fixation space, we innervate not sometimes this and sometimes that muscle through whose action the focusing would be possible, but the same muscles are always innervated in the same way as long as the musculature is not somehow disturbed. The innervation and its corresponding muscle action is a single-valued function of the position of the fixation point in fixation space.

This arrangement, which the following will prove, is of great importance for mastering eye movements because with it the necessary innervation for every given position and motion of the point of fixation is inalterably determined. If fixation were, for instance, sometimes held in position *P* by one muscle group and sometimes by another, and was then to be moved from *P* in a given direction, the necessary innervation would be dependent on the already present tension and position of the muscles, and the will so to say would have to take this into account in order to accomplish the proposed movement. But if the same position of fixation always implied the same muscle action, the same movement of fixation would also always imply the same change of this action. We need not select the appropriate innervation for every special case, but only to know it once and for all.

To develop this further, if we want to move the fixation point from its given position *P* in a specified direction along a line, it is possible *a priori* that the muscles which we would call into action could mediate only part of this straight line motion of the fixation point in a given direction, so that we would have to call upon other muscles for help, which we might finally have to change again. In reality this is not so. *Rather, the same muscles which begin a movement of the fixation point in a given direction are adequate to continue the movement to the border of the smaller fixation space.* (I define the smaller fixation space of the double eye as that part of the entire larger fixation space which is used exclusively in ordinary vision, because we avoid all strenuous positions by turning the head.)

Even if the same muscles are adequate to describe a straight line of any desired length in fixation space, it would still be conceivable that these muscles are not taking part in the movement with the same antagonistic relationships of powers throughout the whole movement. At the beginning one would be active to greatest advantage while later another must develop the greatest power to hold the fixation point in the prescribed path. This too is not the case. *Rather, if the fixation point is moved through the smaller fixation space in any given straight line, not only are the same muscles active, but these muscles are also active in constant power relationships during the entire execution of the movement. The relative strengths with which the relevant muscles are innervated at the beginning of the movement can therefore remain unchanged throughout the entire movement, and only the absolute strength of innervation need be increased.*

From any given point in the smaller fixation space, fixation can be moved in a direction described by corresponding parallel lines. If fixation were moved in one case from point P in the fixation space along the straight line L and in the other case from the point P' along a line L' parallel to the first, that is, in both cases in the same direction, it would be possible that each case would be executed with different muscles, or if with the same muscles, with a different participation of these muscles. This too is not in fact true. *Rather, the musculature of the double eye and its automatic control (Selbststeuerung) is so arranged that not only do the same muscles always move fixation from any given point in the smaller fixation space in the same direction, but that not even a change in the relationships of the power with which the single muscles take part in the movement is necessary.* Thus the same innervation through which fixation is moved from point P in a given direction also moves it from any other point of the smaller fixation space in the same direction to the borders of the smaller fixation space, and sometimes beyond it; one and the same given innervation of the double eye describes all parallel paths of a given direction in the smaller visual space. Innervation therefore is dependent only on the direction in which movement should occur, and is independent of the point from which it should begin. In other words, *the type of innervation necessary to move the gaze in a given direction is a function only of the direction of this path and not of the position of the path in fixation space.* Only the strength of this innervation and the strength of the muscle contraction corresponding to it must be variable. Proofs for these statements follow later.

In the previous paragraphs it was shown that spatial conceptions direct the movements of the double eye in seeing, and especially that the direction in which the goal point of the movement appears relative to the present fixation point determines the direction of the movement. Correspondingly, we found that we are much more confident of this direction than of the absolute distance of the two points in question from one another or of their position and distance relative to our body. Now if, as was just indicated, the innervation necessary for a given movement of the point of sight depends only on the direction of the goal point of the movement relative to the present point of sight, then an accurate grasp of this direction is a condition of the proper innervation, while knowledge of the other parameters of the two points in fixation space is not necessary to generate the appropriate innervation. Whenever the length of the path from one point to the other has been under or overestimated, the gaze will still find its goal if it has begun on the correct path.

The described arrangement therefore makes it possible for the spatial perceptions which we have with the greatest confidence, namely perceptions of the direction from one point to another, to be given quite directly as the directors of eye movement. If a correct grasp of the absolute positions of objects, an exact estimate of their distances, and an exact determination of their distances from our body were necessary, then the exactness of our eye movements would be significantly reduced by the continual illusions which we suffer in this respect, which will be discussed later. Eye movements would be an important aid for orientation on the form and position of objects if the direction of one point relative to another were adequate for directing them confidently. They could not hope to do this if they could not be directed so simply.

We would need to learn specific innervations through long practice for every position of the double eye if we had to figure the present position of the double eye for every new innervation. We would have to choose a corresponding new innervation in order to move the gaze even further to the left, for instance, if the double eye required different innervations depending upon the present position. If the direction in which the point of sight moved through space determined the type of innervation, independent of its position in visual space, we could give the correct impulse for movement from every point of visual space if we could do it from only one point in visual space.

Visual fixation can move from one point in a straight line in as many radiating directions as one can imagine, and each direction expresses a special manner or, so to say, coloring of the innervation necessary to fulfill the movement. Since the beginning point of the movement can assume any position in visual space, the number of these types of innervation is not increased.

Everyone is accustomed to a special posture of the hand during writing; if he changes it, the script changes its appearance, though it indeed retains certain individual characteristics. This is clear if one holds his pen at an unaccustomed position relative to the paper during writing, so that it approaches the paper at a different angle. The letters will then immediately become steeper or more angled, and if one attempts to maintain the exact angle and form as usual in spite of the abnormal pen position, there is great effort and incomplete success. If we were now forced for some reason to constantly change the position of the hand and pen, for instance because the paper and with it its lines were turning under the hand, a constant handwriting would obviously be extraordinarily difficult if not impossible. One would find oneself in an analogous position if a special innervation for the movement of the eye was necessary from each individual position. The mechanism of the eye is thus more comfortably arranged in this respect than that of the hand. The lines which the hand writes on the paper appear very different in spite of a constant intention and innervation, depending upon how the pen or such lies on the paper. But vision always describes the same lines of figures in visual space with the same intentions and innervations, whether or not it has this or that position of the line of sight.

9. *The Basic Law of Innervation and Muscle Action*

Each of the three main dimensions of space corresponds to two special muscle groups of the double eye which serve to move the fixation point in two opposite directions (see below). We therefore have six muscle groups to differentiate, each of which can be handled by the will so to say as a single muscle. Elsewhere in the organism many muscles are so related to one another for common function that a single stimulus releases a simultaneous action of the whole group, whereby the degree of participation of each single muscle with respect to the others is determined in advance. In sneezing, for instance, a single stimulus sets a whole group of muscles into actions already determined in strength and timing. In the same way specific eye muscles respond to a single impulse of will in a coordinated way according to the relative and previously determined allotments of the single muscles.

If we hold the head erect, two of the six muscle groups provide movement in the dimension of breadth; one which I will call the group of *right-turners* directs the point of vision of the double eye horizontally to the right while the other, the *left-turners,* directs it horizontally to the left from whichever point in visual space the movement originates. A second double group, the *raisers* and *lowerers,* provides vertical movements; one deviates the fixation of the double eye from any position upward and the other downward. Two final groups mediate movement in the direction of depth, one bringing the point of sight further from and the other nearer to the head; the first group could be called the *out-turners* or *abductors* and the latter, the *in-turners* or *adductors.*

For all other directions of movement, two or three muscle groups combine for common action. According to the relationships of powers with which the single groups here participate, the results of the common action fall in various directions. For instance, if the right-turners and the raisers are simultaneously active, fixation moves to the right and up, and the steeper its path, the greater the pulling power of the raisers is in comparison to that of the right-turners. If action of the adductors is added to these two groups, the fixation point simultaneously comes closer to the face.

The group of right-turners of the double eye consists of the right lateral rectus and the left medial rectus, and the left-turners are the left lateral rectus and the right medial rectus. The two medial recti constitute principally the group of adductors and the two lateral recti, the abductors. (We will see below that innervation for the purpose of bringing the fixation point nearer involves not only the two medial recti, but also and simultaneously the intraocular muscles which move the iris and those which accomplish accommodation for nearness, as well as still other extraocular muscles, so that here too a large number of muscles is associated. For the time being, in the interest of simplicity, I will ignore these and limit myself to consideration of the innervation of the two medial recti necessary for bringing the fixation point nearer.) We find that each of the four muscles named is a part of two groups; for instance, the left medial rectus is sometimes linked with the lateral and sometimes with the medial rectus of the right eye for common action. We frequently see analogous relationships, be they inborn or acquired, in the organism. Coughing as well as sneezing rests upon an inborn arrangement of linkages of many muscles for common action. The muscles which mediate sneezing are not entirely the same as those which mediate coughing, but rather only certain ones and specifically the breathing muscles partake in both actions; others, such as certain gum muscles, participate only in sneezing while still others, for instance certain larynx muscles, act only in coughing. These breathing muscles behave similarly to the eye muscles named above in that they function sometimes as part of one muscle association and sometimes another. There are numerous examples of this.

The groups of raisers and lowerers consist of four muscles each; the two superior recti and the two inferior obliques constitute the group of raisers, while the two inferior recti and the two superior obliques are the group of lowerers of the double eye.

By this analysis we need control, so to say, only six motors in vision. The goal of seeing clearly an object exactly above the presently fixated point, for instance, requires an innervation of the motor which moves the point of sight upward. That this motor consists of four divisions, the four muscles of the raising group, is as irrelevant as the number of gears constituting a machine, as long as it obeys the machine operator's intentions.

As has already been explained, the described functions of the six muscle groups are the same no matter what the starting point of the movement in visual space. The muscles of the two eyes are controlled such that one and the same innervation of the same muscles always drives the same relative fixation change with every eye movement in spite of the change of position of the muscle insertions on the bulb. In order to raise the fixation point, for instance, one and the same innervation of the raiser group specified above is adequate whether the fixation point was higher or lower, left or right, in visual space at the beginning of the movement.

Consider as a visual field a very distant plane parallel to the facial surface, and on it, lying exactly opposite the face, a vertical and a horizontal line. The vertical deviation of any fixated point on this plane from the horizontal line is a measure of raising or lowering; the horizontal deviation from the vertical line measures the right or left turning of fixation. Now, in order to raise the fixation from the horizontal midline of this visual field and to direct it upward for a given distance, an always equal *quantity* and equal *type* of innervation is adequate no matter from which point on the horizontal midline the raising began, and similarly, an always equal innervation of the lowerers is adequate to move the fixation from the horizontal for a given distance downward. Only for the peripheral parts of the field of vision is this no longer exactly true. If we have further raised fixation a specific distance over the horizontal midline and now want to let it glide to the right, it is adequate to let the already present innervation of the raisers remain unchanged and to introduce innervation of the right turners; the former hold the fixation always at the same height while the latter push it horizontally to the right no matter how much the horizontal path of fixation deviates from the middle horizontal.

In like manner if fixation were turned to the right at the beginning and should now be raised, it would be adequate to hold the already existing innervation of the right turners unchanged and to innervate the raisers in addition: fixation would rise vertically independent of how far to the right its path deviated from the vertical midline, if only it is not too near the borders of the binocular visual field.

To remain with our example, if a point *P* is given in the upper right quadrant of the visual field, the vertical deviation of this point from the middle horizontal corresponds to a specific strength of raising innervation, and its sideward deviation to the right of the middle vertical line to a specific degree of innervation of the right turners. The relationship of the intensities of these two innervations corresponds to the relationship between the height and the sideward deviation of the fixated point. The two innervations are carried out on the corresponding muscles whether simultaneously or sequentially and whether the innervation for raising occurs before sideward deviation, or vice versa: in every case fixation will come to lie on the same point of the visual field. If fixation found itself, therefore, in the middle of the field of vision and should now be moved to the given point *P*, that is, obliquely right and upward, one has only to let the two innervations occur simultaneously in the specified relationships of strength in order to reach the goal.

If I thus used two muscle groups innervated with varying relationships of intensity, I could move fixation from its middle position in any direction in the field of vision. But to move fixation from a deviated position in a given straight or oblique direction, I need only to maintain the innervation corresponding to the already existing deviation of fixation and to add to it the innervation necessary to move fixation from the middle position in the same direction, that is, to move it parallel to the required direction.

If fixation is raised and is to be lowered again, a simple release of the ongoing raising innervation would be adequate for a lowering to the midline; further lowering would then require still another innervation of the lowering muscles. In reality the latter innervation indeed appears to occur immediately, while the original innervation of the raisers gradually disappears. What applies to these two antagonistic muscle groups can be transposed to all other cases in which fixation is transferred from one quadrant of the visual field to another.

Finally we have still to consider that the fixation point also moves in the dimension of depth and is moved toward or away from the face. If we consider a fixation point *A* in the median plane before us, and lying not too far away in a plane parallel to the facial plane, then this plane divides visual space into front (nearer) and back (further) halves. The median plane itself divides it into left and right, and the plane of fixation into upper and lower halves. Now the direction in which a second point *B* lies relative to point *A* can be specified by the relationship of its deviations from the three given planes, and from that we know its direction if we know how far point *B* lies over or under the fixation plane, right or left from the median plane, and in front of or behind the vertical plane parallel to the face. The direction in which point *B appears* to lie relative to the fixation point *A* will correspond approximately to the *true* direction in normal vision. If we have grasped this direction, we have simultaneously grasped the relationships of deviations of the point *B* from the three planes intersecting at the fixation point *A*, and we now need only to innervate the three corresponding muscle groups in the same relationships to move fixation from *A* to *B*. Thus if point *B* appears to us equally higher and nearer and further to the right than the fixated point *A*, we must innervate the raisers, the right turners and the adductors all equally strongly to bring the fixation successfully to *B*. But if the vertical deviation of point *B* appears to exceed the deviation to the side and in nearness, we must innervate the raisers correspondingly more strongly than the other two muscle groups, and so forth. Had we already raised or lowered the double eye in order to fixate the point *A* or moved to the right or left, it would be the same as if we had raised or lowered the entire head or turned it right or left. We could then read off the innervations necessary for a given movement of fixation in the same way as before, if we only remember that the same innervation which was necessary to focus the double eye on the first point A will always be thought of as maintained, and that giving up or putting aside the already existing innervation of a muscle group will have the same result as a newly applied innervation of the antagonsitic group.

These arrangements, in which the type of innervation appears to depend only on the direction of the prospective fixation movement, reveal very simple innervation relationships in comparison to the inexhaustible variety of movement. Through the arrangements just described, these are simplified even more. The supervision and direction of the single muscles is spared. Because each of the six described muscle groups is innervated as a whole, each of the three double groups corresponds to one of the three dimensions to which we want to orient in visual space, and the innervation approaches exactly the perception of space. The motor functions of the double eye then originate even more clearly in beautiful harmony with their sensory functions. Our understanding of space is indeed very uncertain in many ways, but even with the first look into a still unknown visual space, we are, with upright heads, fairly confidently informed about what is positioned vertically, what is at equal heights, that is, horizontally, and what is at equal nearness or distance, even if we suffer numerous confusions about absolute position. This is especially true if we have not yet explored the space with the help of eye movements. We orient ourselves most easily on the three main dimensions, and with this the appropriate grasp of the relative deviations of one point from another on these three dimensions is possible, that is, the grasp of the direction of one point relative to another. With the grasp of this direction we are also given immediately which muscle groups we must innervate and in which relationships of strength.

Of course the law of innervation and muscle actions discussed here is not carried through with mathematical exactness. In fact, there are many small deviations, especially in the more pheripheral parts of visual space, to which a special discussion will be dedicated (Ch. 11 – B.B.).

With eye movements the insertions of the eye muscles on the eyeball change their position with respect to the orbital insertion, and consequently the pulling direction of the contracting muscle as well as its antagonist can also change. Therefore a certain automatic control must be arranged if the eye is indeed to respond with the same movements to one and the same innervation in spite of varying initial positions. We will find that the regulation of the eye muscles is such that nothing contradicts the assumptions made above, and from purely mechanical considerations it is most unlikely that innervations intended for relatively similar fixation movements are influenced by the present fixation position and its corresponding innervation.

Following Helmholtz's view, one must assume that not only the present fixation position of the double eye but even the position of each individual eye is somehow relevant in consciousness. These must be figured into the innervation if one wants to explain the lawfulness with which the eyes move, especially in regard to the cyclorotary position of the retina to be discussed later. Helmholtz considers each eye as a movement organ which originally is fully independent. He must therefore assume, for instance, that both medial recti and both lateral recti are innervated to a different degree in unsymmetrical convergence focusing, so that just to somehow displace the point of fixation, and not even considering the cyclorotary orientation of the retina, each eye would require a special innervation. This assumption has already been disproved by the above proof for the inborn relationship of both eyes.

10. *Proofs for the Law of Innervation*

The validity of the law of innervation expressed in the above paragraphs can be derived with great likelihood simply from the arrangement of the eye muscles, but for closely related reasons it cannot be rigorously proved. To do this a mathematically exact knowledge of the modes of operation of the single muscles and the resistances which oppose each single movement would be necessary. The great simplicity of this law, the easy overview which it gives us over the apparently so complex coordination of the various muscles, and the clear harmony which it establishes between the sensory and motor functions of the organ of sight cannot be compelling grounds for its validity. The necessity for recognizing it as correct lies for me much more in the following considerations.

As already mentioned in chapter 5, the eye movements may not be thrown together with the pure reflex movements, though I hold it to be appropriate to make certain analogies with the latter. Those who have performed any experiments in this area will know how much eye movements give the impression of being involuntary in countless cases, as an indirectly seen retinal image so to say pulls the eye to its side against our will. One should remember the power with which indirectly seen mouches volantes ("fleeting flies," vitreous floaters) and afterimages force our eyes to move without or against our effort at movement, just as the double images which one frequently experiences with the first look into a stereoscope show the least tendency to resolution when one tries to do this most strongly and moves the eyes on purpose. But the images approach one another by themselves and flow into one another as soon as one leaves the eyes to themselves, etc. All of these phenomena are easy to explain if one assumes an inborn or extensively practiced relationship between the retinal position on one hand, on which the indirectly seen image lies, and the innervation on the other hand which is necessary to move this image to the center of the retina; in other words, if one therefore assumes that the position of the indirect image on the retina is simultaneously the determining factor for the necessary innervation.

In fact, such a relationship is frequently assumed without the consequences of the assumption, which are nothing further than the recognition of the innervation law described above.

As soon as one assumes the contrary, that now one and now another innervation is necessary for similar movement of fixation according to the already existing fixation position and eye focus, i.e., *that the same displacement of an image on the retina must be accomplished now through one and now through another innervation,* then the innervation necessary to transfer the indirect image to

the center of the retina is no longer a function of the position of the image but is simultaneously a function of the present eye position, and there is no longer any question of a parallel between eye movement and reflex movement. Language also has a parallel with reflex movement insofar as a thought or a read word immediately leads by reflex to the movements necessary for its pronounciation. Assume now that the innervation necessary for this is dependent upon the present head position, that one must innervate different muscles or the same muscles in other ways in order to pronounce the same word when the head is nodding forward. This relationship is analogous to that assumed by those who make the innervation of the eyes dependent on the present position of fixation or, in other words, on the present position of the head relative to the objects of sight.

Further, the law of equal innervation of both eyes whose validity was proven above is unthinkable without the law of muscle action just discussed. The coordination of eye movements demands one and the same innervation for both eyes. If fixation is raised vertically with unsymmetrical eye position, however, then the right eye needs a different innervation from the left because the line of sight of the right eye makes a different angle with the median plane than the left; thus each eye would have to be innervated for itself. If to turn fixation horizontally to the left, innervation had to take into account the angle about which each eye is already deviated inward or outward, or if the medial or lateral rectus could not accomplish the movement to the right or left under all circumstances, then an equal and simultaneous innervation of both eyes would only exceptionally accomplish its goal; in the great majority of cases each eye would have to be innervated differently.

Consider that the muscles of both eyes are arranged symmetrically so that one muscle system is the mirror image of the other, though symmetrical movements are indeed relatively uncommon and most of them by far are asymmetrical. Symmetrical movements in which both lines of sight intersect only in a median plane can, or course, be accomplished only by equal innervation of muscles of the same name in both eyes. But in reality, even simple cases of vision with parallel lines of sight concern only asymmetrical positions and movements inasmuch as the lines of sight are not parallel to the median plane. Here the direction of the double eye by simple innervation is conceivable only if the symmetrical arrangement of the muscles of the two eyes is made, so to say, so innocuous that the two raisers and the two lowerers each function as one muscle which raises or lowers fixation under all circumstances. Thereby the two muscle systems, although they are symmetrical in form, would function as a

single system and not as two bilaterally symmetrical ones, and it is now obvious that congruent as well as symmetrical movements of both eyes can be produced by a single innervation.

If the innervation necessary for relatively similar movements of fixation were a function of the present eye position, the position of the point of sight would always have to be in our consciousness in order, so to say, to figure it into the innervation. But if it were always present it would have to betray itself, it seems to me, through an exact localization of the presently fixated object. Now the latter is not the case; rather, the grossest confusions about the position of the point of sight occur frequently and the localization of the fixated object is always most uncertain if we have no other reference points for the judgement of position. Now in such cases where we localize the point of sight falsely we should expect to choose a particular innervation for the purpose of a given fixation movement. This would not be adapted to the real but to the intended fixation position, if another innervation with another fixation position were necessary for relatively the same movement. But this false innervation would result in a movement of the eye which must be differentiated from that which would occur with proper innervation. This difference would not reveal itself by a false movement of the point of sight, which finds its goal under all circumstances, because the latter is visible to us and with this we can correct the deviation of fixation from the intended path with another further innervation. The false innervation, however, would indeed determine another orientation of the retina which would have to be detectable if it were in any way significant. But as can be shown, the orientation of the retinas is always the same with one and the same movement of the point of sight, whether we localize the latter correctly or falsely. This speaks for the assumption that confusions over the position of the point of sight do not disturb the lawful mastery of eye movements, because these movements are directed by innervations which are independent of the present fixation position.

11. *Deviations from the Laws of Muscle Actions Described in Chapter 9*

I have already mentioned in passing that the operation of the six described muscle groups is not always exactly the same, as the above schema assumes. Many small but important deviations will be pointed out later. Here it will suffice to discuss only the most important and at the same time to determine to what degree new proofs for the already given laws of innervation can be found in these deviations.

I should first note that the action of the muscle group defined above as raisers does not move the line of sight vertically upward when working alone, but also moves somewhat outward, while the group of lowerers does not pull directly downward but simultaneously somewhat inward. Now because we innervate only the raisers or lowerers when we want to raise or lower fixation in the vertical direction, it follows that these muscles do not correctly carry out our will, but that without or rather against our will an inward or outward deviation of the lines of sight from the vertical path occurs.

In a later section the visual disturbances which follow from this involuntary deviation of the eye will be discussed. There it will be shown that we generally localize the retinal image of the fixated point where we had intended to position the point of sight. If our muscles do not correctly carry out this intention, a confusion over the position of the fixated object results. As I will show, such a confusion also occurs as a result of the above deviations, if one must specify only with the help of eye movements what is positioned vertically above or below.

It is known that lowering the visual plane promotes an increase in the convergence angle of the lines of sight, while raising tends to reduce it. Helmholtz (13) explains this by saying that we have become accustomed to linking a lowering of fixation with a simultaneously greater convergence because this aids in seeing distant objects with a raised visual plane and near objects with a lowered one. I do not hold this explanation to be correct because other further effects show that this phenomenon is grounded in the mechanism of the musculature, and that the convergence which occurs with lowering of the visual plane is not voluntarily learned but enters in involuntarily for purely mechanical reasons. If it were learned for the purpose of near vision, the focusing muscles would be innervated together with the innervation of the medial recti and the convergence implied by lowering of the visual plane would be linked to a corresponding accommodation for nearness. Such an effect does not occur, as will be shown in Part Four; rather, the eyes converge without changing their focal condition, while the latter is always changed as soon as convergence is voluntarily increased for the purpose of near vision.

This proves, therefore, that convergence with lowering of the visual plane is determined not by a simultaneously occurring habitual innervation of the medial recti but purely mechanically through the arrangement of the musculature, and this indeed appears to be the reason for the peculiar insertion of the obliques as they lie on the upper and lower edges of the eyeball. Even so, the symptoms of pareses and paralyses of the lateral recti show that the latter exhibit smaller resistance to their function with a raised visual plane than with a lowered one, and that their working range is not divided from that of the medial recti by a vertical border but by one which is somewhat slanted outward above and inward below.

The lateral and medial recti also do not move fixation exactly horizontally when they are operating alone, for here too deviations from the intended horizontal movement occur. These, however, are much smaller than those described above. In general, the medial rectus simultaneously turns fixation slightly downward and the lateral rectus upward. I will return to this later.

With strong raising or lowering of fixation, one line of sight often remains behind downward or upward with respect to the other. If I turn my parallel lines of sight to the right with a strongly raised visual plane and upright head, my right line of sight deviates downward. If this deviation is small, it will be corrected by a small one-sided innervation of the raiser of the right eye, as we have seen in chapter 5 with the prism experiments. But because one can innervate the muscle groups of one eye more strongly than the corresponding ones of the other eye only within very narrow limits, this correction very soon becomes impossible as the deviation of the right line of sight increases downward with strong right turning of fixation. Double images over one another occur immediately. This is not because it is mechanically impossible for the right eye to raise itself so strongly, for the focus of the right line of sight at the desired height succeeds if I close the left eye without moving the head. I can prove this more than adequately because an afterimage created in the retinal center of the right eye appears on the intended object. Rather, the reason for this phenomenon is that due to increased resistances of the right eye, which is strongly turned outward, the raisers cannot pull as hard with equally strong innervation as the raisers of the left eye which is turned inward. Thus we have in the facts described a further proof for the law of equal innervation of both eyes. For if the raisers of the right eye could be innervated very much more strongly than those on the left at the same time, the double images could not appear.

My right eye, in turning to the right with raised fixation, behaves in the same way as my left in turning to the left. Of course, many

individual characteristics come into play here according to the movement of the eyeball because of its gestalt, or the form of the orbits, or if larger resistances occur in this or that direction for other reasons. With each paresis of the eye muscles analogous phenomena occur in instructive ways and prove the innervation laws given above.

Many fixation positions show a certain holding back of one line of sight inward or outward even before the line of sight comes to the end of its range, if the *side-by-side* double images thus created cannot be united again by a small innervation of the adductor or abductor groups.

Therefore, we may not consider the law of muscle actions just described as mathematically exactly fulfilled, for it is only *a schema which approaches reality very closely.* Small deviations can be corrected easily in the indicated ways and do not lead to noticeable confusions of sight; larger deviations can bring on double vision or noticeable confusions about the location of events.

12. *On the Fixation Space of the Double Eye*

I define the *fixation space of the double eye* as the sum of points which can be fixated binocularly with one and the same head position. The fixation space is therefore to be thought of as bound fast to the head; it changes its position in absolute space only when the head moves.

Fixation space must be differentiated from the *range of the line of sight,* that is, the sum of the lines with which the line of sight can coincide given one and the same head position. These lines, also to be thought of as a space bound fast to the head, describe a cone whose point lies at the turning point of each respective eye. It can be best determined in the following way:

After one has positioned the lines of sight horizontally and parallel straight ahead, one gives the head that tilt from the horizontal by which the fixation plane assumes the so-called primary position, which will be characterized later. In general, the head will then have the accustomed nearly upright position. Then the head will be fixed by a method to be described later (chapter 16). Parallel to the lines connecting the nodal points, a vertical glass pane will be erected and marked with thick ink or oil paint where the horizontal lines of sight (in the primary position) intersect the glass. Behind the glass pane a small disk is erected with a color approximately complementary to the colored background, on a wall as far away as possible for those with normal vision, and for the short-sighted at the far point of their eyes. This disk will be fixed so that one receives a lasting afterimage of it. One then lets the fixation wander on the distant wall in any direction until it can go no further and lets the afterimage stand on the wall. At this moment one marks the glass pane at the point where the line of sight intersects it. Then one turns back to the colored disk, refreshes the afterimage again and lets the line of sight wander in another direction to the border of its range, etc. In this way one constructs a row of points on the glass pane which one connects into a curve representing the vertical cross section of the conical surface which borders the range of the line of sight. After one has constructed this curve for both eyes, the angle about which the lines of sight can deviate in any given direction from the primary position can be found from the curves and from the distance of the glass pane from the point of rotation of the eyes. The afterimage is indispensible because there is otherwise no control over whether the line of sight really lies on the point which one believes to be fixated; confusion in this respect is very easy with strong turning of the eyes.

The angles through which my line of sight can turn from the primary position in the vertical and horizontal directions are the following:

	left eye	*right eye*
1. upward	20°	20°
2. downward	62°	59°
3. inward	44°	46°
4. outward	43°	43°

According to Donders, the average excursion distances of the lines of sight of the normal eye are: inward, 45 degrees; outward, 42 degrees; upward, 34 degrees; and downward, 47 degrees. But here the primary position is not taken as the middle position.

The curves drawn on the glass pane are shown reduced in figure 4. The broken line represents the right and the solid line the left eye. The line *ab* shows the distance from the pane of glass to the rotation points on the same scale, while *l* and *r* are the points where the left and right lines of sight intersect the glass pane in the primary position. The curve of the coutour of the nose is represented inward and downward. The range of my line of sight therefore has the following horizontal or vertical diameters of opening angle (going through the primary position):

	left eye	*right eye*
1. horizontal	87°	89°
2. vertical	82°	79°

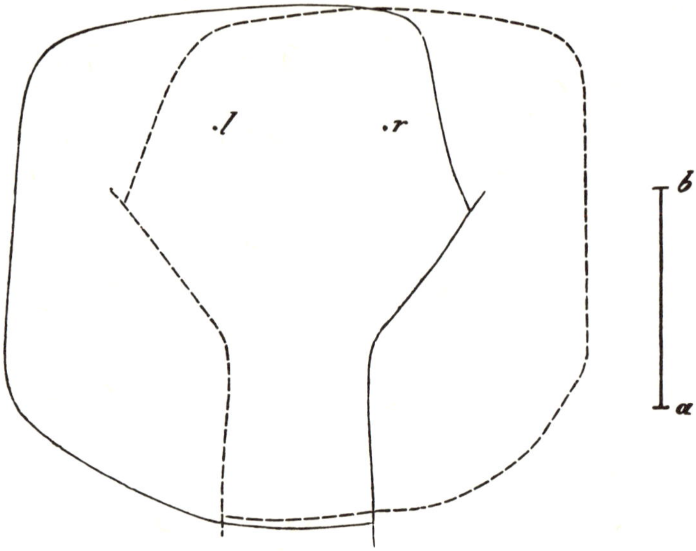

Fig. 4.

If I consider a plane vertical to the primary position of the lines of sight and very distant, and indicate on it the area over which the lines of sight can move, the two monocular fixation fields have the form shown to the same scale in Fig. 5.

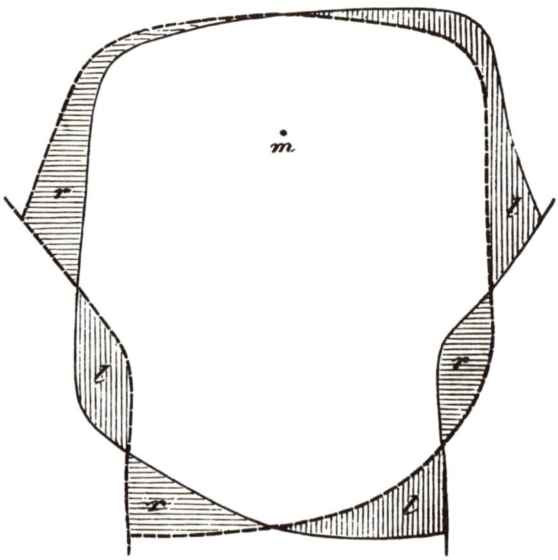

Fig. 5.

The points r and l (Fig. 4) are here superimposed on one point m which represents a very distant fixation point. The figure shows that one eye can be focused on points which the other eye cannot fixate: the two monocular fixation fields do not coincide. The parts on which only the left eye can fixate are vertically striped and are labelled l, while the corresponding areas for the right eye are horizontally striped and are labelled r. The part of the field which is accessible to both eyes (which both monocular fields therefore cover) is not simultaneously accessible to both lines of sight in all parts, as one might think. The vertical binocular fixation field conceived at a great distance is much more limited. In Fig. 6, I have shown this binocular fixation field of the double eye looking at a distance, to the same scale shown in the field which is accessible with monocular vision. For my eyes it lies not quite symmetrically about the median plane, because my two eyes do not behave quite equally in their motility.

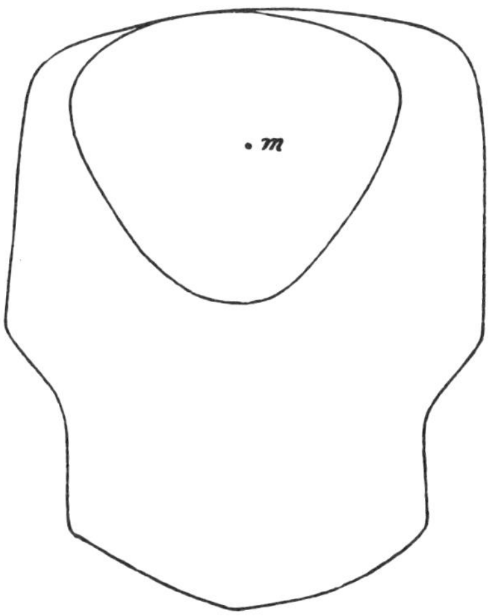

Fig. 6.

This reduction of the binocular fixation field in comparison with the common areas of the two monocular fields can be explained in the following way: we are not able to innervate the abductors of the double eye as strongly as we can the other five muscle groups. This is already revealed because diverging squint cannot be learned in spite of long practice at it, as can convergence. After years of practice I myself have only reached the stage where I can diverge nearly five degrees with strongly raised visual plane of the lines of sight. It is not known to me whether anyone can voluntarily diverge more strongly. If I give myself the task of alternating my binocular fixation from a far to a near point in quick succession, I need a much shorter time to transfer fixation from the far to the near point than I do from the near to the far. It almost gives me the impression that the two lines of sight in the latter case separate only because the innervation of the medial recti ceases, but not because the lateral recti are innervated. In any case, the return of the lines of sight to parallelism is primarily grounded in the effort of the musculature to restore the balance of elastic forces, that is, to bring the eyeball back into the resting position, and only slightly in the weak activity of the lateral recti which we can voluntarily produce. If we lower the parallel lines of sight they begin involuntarily to converge for purely mechanical reasons, as was mentioned in the above chapters. As long as this convergence is very small, we can correct it through the weak innervation of the abductor group which is possible for us, but with increasing lowering of the visual plane this innervation is no longer adequate, and then parallel positioning of the lines of sight is no longer possible; thus the restriction of the binocular field of fixation occurs with distant vision downward.

If I turn the far-accommodated double eye to the right or the left by innervation of the sideward turners, then one medial rectus and one lateral rectus receives an equally strong innervation. But with stronger sideward turning the power of the lateral rectus lags behind that of the medial, either because it must overcome greater resistances or because it is a weaker muscle than the medial rectus. This also shows that the excursion distance of my eyes is somewhat smaller outward than inward. The outward turned eye therefore remains somewhat behind the inward turned one as soon as the innervation of the abductor group which is possible for me is no longer adequate for correction of the deviation; this explains the relative restriction of the binocular fixation field to the left and right with distance vision.

It is the same with near vision as with far vision: the binocular fixation space has much narrower limits than one might expect from the excursion ability of the eyes. One need only move a small object around near the face and follow it with the eyes, and it will already be seen double even when it is still significantly far from the borders of the region common to the range of both lines of sight, that is, in a position where each eye can still fixate comfortably. If with raised fixation plane, one brings an object lying in the median plane so near that binocular fixation of it is difficult and brings forth the feeling of strong effort from the eye, and then closes one eye, he will note that it requires no effort at all to focus the line of sight of the open eye on the object, and it does not matter which eye is the open one. The object breaks down into unsymmetrical double images if it is brought even closer, although even here the line of sight of each single eye can be focused on it as soon as the other eye is closed. Thus, we can move the single eye more strongly inward by innervating the side turners than we can by innervating the adductors to bring the point of sight nearer. It may be that the latter innervation cannot be accomplished with the same strength as the former, but it may also be that the inward turning encounters larger resistances in one case than the other, which is not impossible because with one and the same deviation of the line of sight inward, the eye is under the influence of different muscle activations for far and near vision (as will be shown in chapter 19).

Of course, the statements made here about fixation space have individual value only in defining the form of fixation space, and they are generally valid to the degree that they relate to causes which reduce the binocular fixation space in comparison to the monocular. Eyes in which the dominance of the medial recti over the lateral recti is smaller than with mine will have a relatively larger binocular fixation space.

Hering's Law summarizes his most important contribution to oculomotor control theory. In the first twelve chapters of this book, Hering thoroughly puts forward this idea and documents it with a variety of thought-provoking, careful and exciting experiments.

Hering's Law first states that "the double eye is a single organ." Equal controlling innervations to corresponding muscles, analogous to single reins to a pair of horses, tightly link the right and left eyes to form this single organ. Hering's analogy to horses and reins is superior to that of the often used one of yoked pair of oxen; the eyes have *no* mechanical link but rather follow a common control law.

The innate nature of this compulsive linking is an important part of Hering's proposal, and he says elegantly that the evidence for it rests not primarily on logic or theory but most solidly on careful observations of newborns who show conjugate tightly linked eye movements even with one eye covered. Again and again he argues against the Helmholtzian 'learning by association' theory. In addition to putting forward various experimental observations to prove innateness, Hering repeatedly points out that learning may indeed cause minor disassociations of innate reflexes. An example that comes to mind is the arm swing while walking. This appears to be an innate or inborn spinal cord pattern which can be modified and even suppressed.

Hering points out that physical movements in the world of experience are a good source of commands to produce linked innervation and that many phenomena are partly due to selective attention. Helmholtz's famous observations on sleep are re-argued brilliantly to indicate that the inborn linking pattern of the nervous system may indeed be disrupted by sleep, an observation that now has recent data in single-cell oculomotor neurophysiology to support it, related to irregular neural discharge for eye movements during drowsiness or sleep. Open loop, as we now term it, tracking of 'mouche' is also used by Hering to show *fixed* association under unusual eye movement conditions.

In a number of crucial observations, he discusses the sensory world and the cyclopian eye as modified or influenced by dominance of an eye. He further points out that compulsive linking occurs without vision and even when it interferes with vision.

Second, Hering extends the basic law to include binocular coordination for both versional *and* vergence eye movements. He clearly points out that the bifixation point of vision can take on positions within a very wide range but that this does not mean that each eye operates independently. There is an extensive review of the way the eyes move during asymmetrical vergence movements. This of course is the classical proof of Hering's Law, showing that for rapid asymmetrical vergences the eye makes saccades and vergences in such a fashion that one eye often will move away from its target with a saccadic version movement. No explanation other than Hering's Law can account for this crucial and repeatedly confirmed observation.

Part of Hering's discussion concerns the site of cancellation of the version and vergence innervations. Hering brings forth evidence suggesting that the muscles receive increased innervation when driven by both vergence and version controls and that the cancellation occurs by summing the forces involved on the eyeball itself. He noted a 'twitching' of the eyeball and adduced this as evidence for peripheral localization of the summation and cancellation sites. This issue has not yet been fully resolved, though several laboratories are working on this problem (Kenyon and Stark). Breinin was the first to adduce evidence for the validity of Hering's Law, but opted for cancellation at the brain stem level. Hering himself, as we shall see below, provided evidence for the idea that static muscle force is solely a function of eyeball position.

Though Hering thought of vertical vergence as an exception to his Law, we now see this to be another example of the Law. One of the reasons why Hering thought of vertical vergence as an exception was that in limiting his concern with the motivation of eye muscles in the interest of vision to the case of a fixed head, he did not see why vertical vergences should occur at all. There is, however, a common situation in vision calling for vertical vergences. Whenever the head tilts, the vestibular system will quickly compensate by causing an appropriate conjugate cyclorotation, maintaining the orientation of the horizontal axis in each eye. This rotates the two eyes into a state of vertical divergence and requires a compensatory vertical convergence movement so that a horizontal line in the field of view continues to appear as a continuous horizontal line when the visual field is undivided. Vertical vergence, by reducing disparity, thus permits fusion to be maintained.

Next, Hering's Law deals with the complexity of the four muscles involved in vertical eye movements. There is an evolutionary change from the primitive insertion of the obliques that act as cyclorotators in fish to the posterior insertions in man that enable the obliques to act as vertical rotators, together with the vertical recti. Hering states that these four vertical eye muscles act as a single motor; that the innervation to these four must be considered as one innervation (in modern language, they share only one degree of freedom). The existence of a raising system with doubled muscles extends the horizontal range of Hering's "smaller fixation space," in which control signals can be independent of the starting point of a movement.

The six eye muscles receive only horizontal and vertical commands. Hering makes some other strong and innovative statements, including the notion that in oblique movements there is a relative allotment of horizontal and vertical innervations; for all parallel oblique movements the relative allotments are fixed; and both the initial position from which the eye moves and the final position to which the eye moves are irrelevant to the size of the command.

Hering justifies the relative allotment constraint because it represents an appropriate mapping of the motor to the horizontal and vertical sensory system. If the concept of two orthogonal components is a valid part of the oculomotor computational machinery, then this may simply be a requirement of an efferent-copy Frame of Reference computation.

Hering admits to deviations from Hering's Law and points out that the 'overall' double eye fixation space is greater than the 'normal' double eye fixation space. He presents a number of interesting experiments showing that the sum of the monocular eye fixation spaces is greater than the overall double eye fixation space, which in turn is greater than the normal double eye fixation space. He further shows that these spaces are functions of the distance of the binocular point and are strongly limited by vergence movements. Hering agrees with Helmholtz that extreme position causes cyclorotation and points out that viewing upward causes divergence while viewing downward causes convergence.

Dynamic Violations of Hering's Law. Neither Hering nor Helmholtz had much awareness of the dynamic characteristics of eye movements. It was only later in the century that Helmholtz' pupil, Lemansky, using a method related to the afterimage of an oscillating light was able to determine that the peak velocities of eye movements were as high as 1,000° per second. It really waited until Dodge's work at the end of the century to understand that eye movements had different dynamic characteristics, which enabled Dodge to classify them into saccades, smooth pursuits, vergences, and other categories. It is now well known that dynamic violations of Hering's Law are exceedingly common. The right eye and the left eye do not make the same shape saccades when looked at from the point of view of 'hyper-fine structure.' This variability is due to variability in the nonlinear, time optimal, pulse-step neural control signal. A single Hering's Law controller drives two independent saccadic pulse generators.

In addition, oblique movements do not have simultaneous horizontal and vertical components; therefore, oblique trajectories have a wide variety of curves, hooks, angles, and bends, which are monocular rather than binocular. The final position of the double eye after an oblique movement, however, is in conformity with Hering's Law. Therefore one is tempted to restrict Hering's Law to static positions at the end of movements rather than be left with the current situation that dynamic violations of Hering's Law are very common.

A counter example to dynamic violations of Hering's Law is the dynamic adherence to Descartes' Law of Reciprocal Innervation. This means that the saccade, for example, would be most irregular if the antagonist was not shut off by an inhibitory pulse envelope whenever agonist neurons were bursting. Indeed the irregularities in the hyper-fine structure of the saccade leading to dynamic overshoot, overlapping saccades and mismatched glissadic eye movements all follow dynamic trajectories controlled by reciprocal innervation of their agonist and antagonist, as demonstrated by their normal Main Sequence localizations. This raises some important points concerning the anatomical location of the neuron connectivity and interactions which provide for Hering's Law on the one hand and Descartes' Law of Reciprocal Innervation on the other.

Primary and secondary deviations are an example of the working out of Hering's Law of equal and simultaneous innervation of the double eye in spite of a partial paresis of one or more extraocular muscles. When an eye with a paretic muscle is viewing monocularly, the increased innervation required to move the line of sight in the paretic field of gaze is also sent to the covered normal eye, according to Hering's Law. This normal covered eye will therefore move well beyond its conjugate line of sight position. Thus the secondary deviation is very large since it represents movement by normal muscles driven by excessive innervation.

Primary deviation occurs when the normal eye views the target and the paretic eye is the covered eye. According to Hering's Law the linked equal innervation to the paretic muscle does not move it fully to the target, so again the lines of sight are not conjugate and parallel. However, this primary deviation, being the failure of the paretic muscle, is less than the secondary deviation.

The Systems Approach. One cannot help but be struck not only by the intellectual vigor throughout this extraordinary monograph but also by the straightforward acceptance and use of ideas that seem to be of the present century. On a number of occasions Hering adheres in an elegant manner to the systems approach.

A system is a group of phenomena, or a set of mechanisms, that are worthwhile treating in and of themselves for the moment, isolating them from all other interacting systems, although this of course is done knowingly and is not fully justified for other situations. This pragmatic approach also applies to the various levels of analysis and levels of explanation with which one treats a system. One can make cogent arguments at one level of mechanism of a particular system and yet often, perhaps necessarily, be ignorantly wrong or incomplete about system operation at another level. One beautiful example of this is Descartes' Law of Reciprocal Innervation, which is insightful and accurate and has lasted through the centuries as an important work on organization in neural control of movement. At the same time, Descartes' knowledge of the neural conduction process and of the muscle contractile process was incomplete and incorrect; his theory of gas under pressure travelling from brain ventricles through the hollow nerves to muscle is totally wrong.

An example of Hering's important use of the systems approach has to do with his treatment of the vertical musculature of the eyes as one motor. The fact that the motor has four divisions, the vertical recti and the oblique muscles, he says is as irrelevant as the movement of gears in a particular engineering motor. One can measure and utilize the input/output behavior of a motor as a "black box" without dissecting it to see if these important relationships are a function of its motor windings or its output gear train.

Hering's synthesis of vertical eye movements into one motor enabled him to gain great insight and sensitivity in his discussion of vertical eye movements and in his consideration of oblique eye movements. Although he was primarily concerned with the binocular movements of the double eye, his simplifying assumption represented important neurological and physiological constraints which are obeyed by the neurological system for controlling eye movements. The same constraints now appear to underlie such important kinematic principles of monocular movements as Donders' Law and Listing's Law, which are accurate for movements within a modest monocular fixation field. The principle also helps to elucidate the deviations and peculiarities of eye position at large eccentricities from primary position. The eye continues to be controlled as though the signals needed to move it from primary position were still appropriate in spite of changes in effective insertions.

Hering's Insistence on the Experimental Approach

In the controversy between the nativists and the empiricists, which had its roots in philosophy, thinking empiricists on the one hand were often persons who tried to demonstrate things by experiment. The nativists on the other hand emphasized an inborn functionalism of the organism, in some ways related to the vitalist stream of philosophy and religion which of course had important, mostly negative, influences in early pre-evolutionary biology. Thus Helmholtz, as an empiricist and as a brilliant and skilled physiologist and physicist, naturally is expected to be an experimentalist. Hering, being a nativist, is supposed not to be an experimentalist. This is completely incorrect.

The modified nativism of Hering is a strictly non-vitalistic, non-philosophical, scientific attitude, emphasizing the built-in hardware and firmware of the human and animal nervous system. There is nothing mystical about Hering's approach, and he was most sensitive to criticism about himself which exaggerated his point of view.

A striking example of Hering's point of view occurs when he discusses the inborn nature of the neurological linking which has given us that eye movement behavior known as Hering's Law of Equal Innervation. First, he reviews the logical inconsistencies of the arguments made against the inborn nature of the control of eye movements. For example, he points out how one might very well learn a dissociation when the association is inborn. Then he suggests that we put aside these conjectures and arguments from reason and go directly to *observation* of the newborn. He then further points out how one must select newborns with wide-open eyes and with an inclination to attend to a visual target. He observes that the newborn's eye movements are conjugate, that this conjugacy is not due to practice, and that one can observe conjugate movements in the covered eye thus ruling out immediate learning.

Hering uses the example that most movements of the hands are symmetrical, but points out the functional importance of conjugacy in eye movements and then observes that eye movements precede hand movements in ontological development. The conjugacy of eye movements is related to Stark's discovery of the conjugacy of head movements; Descartes' Law of Reciprocal Innervation is a law of the conjugacy of movements of the single eye, a monocular Hering's Law. Two antagonistic muscles act as a pair just as the two eyes act as a pair.

Again and again in this remarkable volume Hering stresses and fully describes marvelous experiments, paying particular attention to the detailed experimental techniques necessary to substantiate his observations.

Part II. On the Orientation of the Double Eye

13. *Mechanical Prerequisites*

For simplicity, the eyeball can be considered as a sphere which can be rotated about an immovable middle point. To determine the position of the sphere it is adequate to give the positions of three* points on it which do not lie on the same diameter, or equivalently, to give the positions of two diameters. In the eye it is best to use first the line of sight for this, which one can assume to go through the point of rotation, and second the diameter which is vertical when the line of sight is directed horizontally straight ahead with an upright head. If we know the positions of these two diameters relative to the orbits or to a coordinate system of the head with any eye position, we have determined the position of the eyeball unambiguously in its socket. It is apparent that knowledge of the position of only one diameter, for instance the line of sight alone, is inadequate, because with the same position of the line of sight the rest of the eye can be thought of in many varied positions, which it would run through one after another if it were rotated around the undisturbed line of sight as an axis.

According to our assumption the axes about which the eye can turn must all go through the center of rotation. But one can think of a sphere as turning in two opposite directions about the same axis. Now to represent both the axis and the direction of turning at the same time, or even to resolve a simple rotational force, one must distinguish the two halves of each axis meeting at the point of rotation as *half axes.* If an observer who is in the extension of one of these half axes sees the spherical surface facing him turning like the hand of a clock, then the half axis in which the observer finds himself is labelled the half axis of rotation (a "left-hand rule" – B.B.). The other half of the axis is then the half axis of the opposite rotation about the same axis.

If the half axis of rotation always remains the same during a rotation, then the rotation occurs about a *stationary* or *permanent axis.* But if the axis of rotation is a different one at each moment of the rotation, one calls it a rotation about *momentary* or *instantaneous axes.* Consider two cones as they are used in stereometric instruction; mount one permanently and roll the second about it so that both tips are always together and the sides are always in contact. One now has an example of rotation about momentary axes. Here the moving cone has only *one* stationary point, at its tip, just as the eye has in its rotations. When it is rolled about the fixed cone, the momentary axes of rotation coincide with the straight lines around which the two conical surfaces contact, and this line is clearly a

*Hering writes "two" here, though undoubtedly "three" is intended. B.B.

different one in each instance. Thus so to say, the axis of rotation moves forth in space and describes the surface of the stationary cone; but it also moves about the rotated cone and describes its surface. If one thinks of the eye socket and of a cone so fastened in it that its tip coincides with the point of rotation of the eye while its base images a part of the surface of the eyeball, and one further considers a second cone fixed on the orbit and with its tip also coinciding with the point of rotation, one can also think of the first cone as rotating about the second, whereby it would take the entire eye with it. In this way rotations of the eyes about momentary axes, which occur frequently in reality, can be made understandable.

One first distinguishes *continuous* and *discontinuous* rotations. Discontinuous means the rotations in which the axis of rotation changes its position in steps, and continuous means that the axis of rotation move steadily or is fixed. The rotation just described on two cones is continuous because the axis of rotation moves through infinitely small angles during infinitely small divisions of time. But if we had rolled two pyramids with any number of sides about one another instead of two cones, the edges of the two pyramids would have functioned as axes of rotation. The two pyramids would then have contacted alternately with two surfaces or two edges, or alternatively with one surface and one edge. In the moments of the rotation when two surfaces of the pyramids contacted, the axis of rotation would appear to spring from one edge to the other because the surface contact can be only momentary if the rotation is not to be interrupted. Thus, an infinitely small time period of rotation here corresponds to a change of location of the axis of rotation about an angle of *finite* size.

Every given continuous or discontinuous rotation about a fixed point may be imagined in this way, imagining developments of conical or pyramidal surfaces, where naturally the form of the surfaces can otherwise have infinite variation.

Certain forces are applied on the surface of the eyeball which try to rotate it. The half axis about which a force tries to rotate is called the *half axis of rotational force.* To illustrate the intensity of rotational force, one should think of a portion of the half axis extending from the center of rotation with its length proportional to the intensity. This gives us simultaneoulsy the half axis as well as the intensity of the rotational force. At the same time this intensity corresponds to the speed with which the force would turn the eye if these rotations could occur without any resistance.

If several forces attempt to rotate the eye simultaneously, that is if several moments of rotation are present at the same time, one can construct the resulting moment of rotation from them in a way similar to the construction of a resultant from several forces working on one point. By its position the resulting moment of rotation then gives us the half axis of the resulting rotational force, and through its length gives us the intensity of the latter.

For this purpose one can consider two simultaneously present moments of rotation as two sides of a parallelogram and construct its diagonal. This is the resulting moment of rotation. If there are three simultaneous moments of rotation, one can first construct the resultant of two of them and finally combine it with the third moment to obtain the resulting moment of all three. Or one can consider the three given moments as three intersecting edges of a parrallelepiped and construct the diagonal for which one end falls on the point of rotation. Thus, in Fig. 7 *af* is the resulting moment of rotation of the three moments *ab, ac* and *ad.* It is clear that in analogous fashion one can also construct resultants from additional simultaneous moments of rotation.

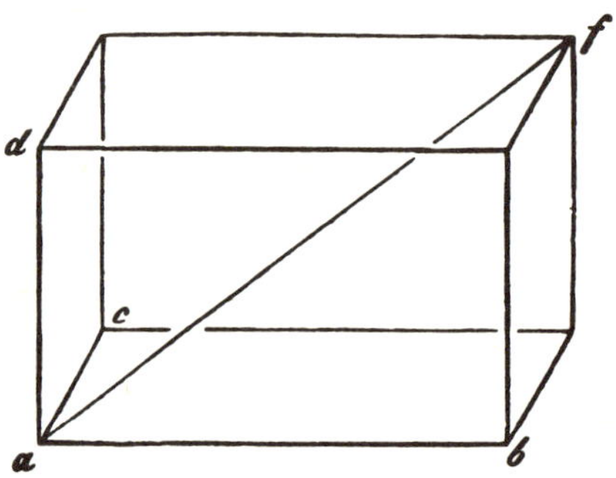

Fig. 7.

Conversely one can interpret each simple moment of rotation as resulting from two or three (or more) simultaneous moments. One then considers these as diagonals of a parallelogram or parallelepiped and constructs the sides or edges necessary for it. The sides or edges which intersect at the point of rotation then represent the moments of rotation into which the given simple moment is analyzed. Because one and the same line can be the diagonal of an infinite number of different parallelograms or parallelepipeds, the analysis of this simple moment is possible in correspondingly many ways.

These then are the rules with which one can find the half axis as well as the size of the resulting rotational force if several forces act simultaneously on the eye. This applies only to an *attempt* at rotation, not to the rotation which actually occurs. The latter will now be considered. Let us take as an example a rotation which occurs under the influence of two simultaneously acting forces.

Given that two forces affect the eyeball simultaneously, one always trying to turn it about a vertical axis in space and the other about a horizontal axis in space, the eye would not turn about either one axis or the other but about the axis of the resulting moment of the two given moments of rotation at each instant. Figure 8 is an equatorial section of the eye from behind, and is perpendicular to the horizontal line of sight through the rotation point of the eye. mv is the half axis about which one force attempts to rotate and mv' is the fixed moment of rotation. If this force alone were active, the line of sight would rotate horizontally to the right. mh is the half axis and mh' the moment of rotation of the other force. If this force alone were active, the line of sight would rotate in a vertical direction downwards. The resulting moment of the two given moments is ms', and ms is thus the half axis about which the true rotation begins and must continue as long as the positions and the relative sizes of the two given moments (and therefore the position of the resulting moment) are not changed.

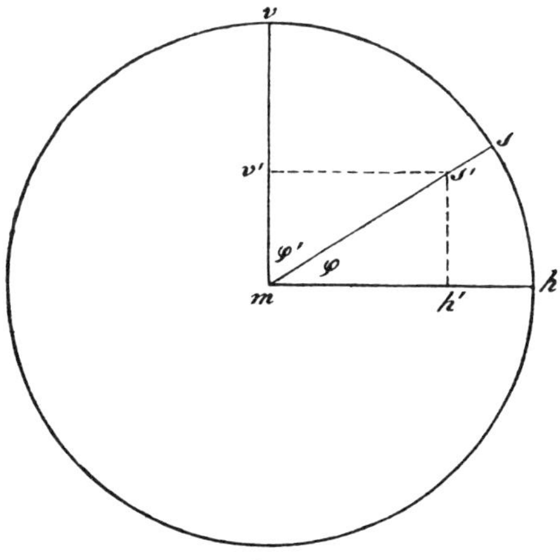

Fig. 8.

Thus when two forces simultaneously try to rotate the eye, and both the position of the half axes and the relationship of size of their two moments of rotation is unchanging, the true rotation occurs about a fixed half axis which lies in the plane of the two given moments of rotation and between them. Specifically, the two angles (φ and φ') which this half axis includes with two moments of rotation of the two forces depend upon the relationships of sizes of the two moments:

$$\tan \varphi = \frac{h's'}{mh'} = \frac{mv'}{mh'}; \qquad \tan \varphi' = \frac{mh'}{mv'}.$$

In the rotation just discussed, the moments of rotation of the two operating forces do not change their positions in space during the course of the rotation, which means that they have thereby changed their positions on the sphere. For the sphere in its rotation about the fixed axis *ms* has rotated relative to the fixed moments of rotation mh' and mv'. We now want to consider the case where the moment of rotation of only one of the two rotating forces contributing to a rotation does not change its position in space, while the other changes its position not on the sphere but in space.

Assume that there were a stiff pin at the location of the line of sight which one could grasp at its free end outside the cornea. One could rotate the eyes in varied ways with this pin. If one simply displaced the free end of the pin, the eye would rotate about an axis perpendicular to the pin and to the direction of its motion. If one rotated the pin between the fingers about itself without displacing it, the eye would be rolled about the line of sight as an axis. But one could also perform both movements simultaneously if one simultaneously activated the two necessary forces, for instance by moving the free end of the pin in a vertical direction downward and simultaneously rotating it about itself between the fingers. Thus the eye would rotate so to say simultaneously about two axes, namely first about the axis at right angles to the line of sight and to its vertical path, that is the horizontal axis, and second about the line of sight itself. While two moments of rotation would be active simultaneously here, the true rotation would occur neither about one axis nor about the other, but its axis would be determined at every moment by the position of the presently *resultant* moment of rotation. But this moment of rotation, and thus also the axis of rotation coinciding with it, would have a different position in space at every instant of the rotation. Specifically, one force continually tries to rotate the eye about the spatially unchangeable horizontal axis *h* while the other wants to rotate it about the line of sight *g*; but the latter changes its position in space during the movement. Thus the plane which contains the moments of rotation of the axes *g* and *h*, and in which the resulting moment of rotation must lie, changes its position at each instant simultaneously with the line of sight by rotating about the axis *h*. For instance, if *mh* in Figure 9 is the horizontal half axis about which one force attempts to rotate the eye downward in a vertical direction, and *mg* is the half axis about which the second force attempts to roll the eye about the line of sight, and if the moment of the first force is twice as great as that of the second, then *mr* represents the moment resulting from *mh'* and *mg'*. If the intensity relationships of the two forces remains the same, the resulting moment will maintain the same position relative to *mh* and *mg* during the entire rotation, with *mh* always at the angle φ and *mg* always at the angle φ'. But the absolute position of the resulting moment *mr* will be a different one at every instant because the line of sight moves downward during the rotation. Now because the rotation at every instant occurs about the half axis in which the resulting moment of rotation lies, the axis of rotation changes its position at every instant. Specifically it describes a circular conical surface in absolute space whose axis coincides with *mh* because it always forms the angle φ with the line *mh*. But in the moving eye it describes a circular conic surface whose axis is *mg* because it always forms the angle φ' with

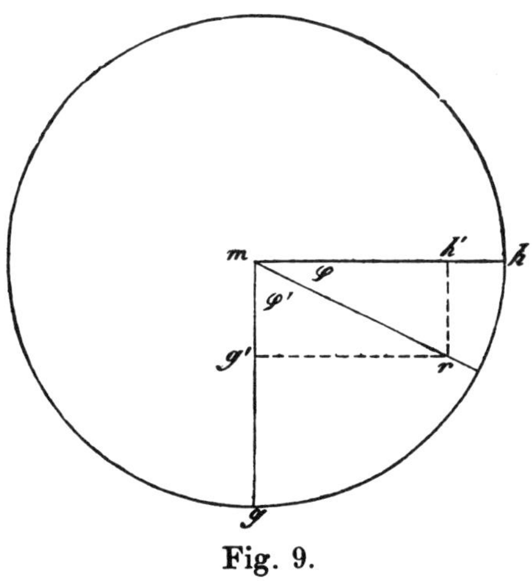

Fig. 9.

the line of sight. These two conical surfaces develop, so to say, around each other during the described rotation. The rotation is thus a continuous one about momentary axes as they were conceived above on the two cones. If the intensity relationships of the two simultaneously active rotation forces were different from what has just been assumed, or if they changed continuously during the rotation, then the path of the momentary rotation axis in absolute space as well as in the sphere would be different, and the conic surfaces which one can think of as developing on one another would have another form. To avoid misunderstanding, I will note here that there are indeed muscles which attempt to rotate the eye about half axes which are at right angles to the line of sight, but there is no muscle which attempts to rotate the eye about the line of sight; thus in reality there are no two muscles which can generate moments of rotation such as we have assumed here.

The above examples show how one rotation results from several simultaneous rotational forces. The resultant occurs about entirely different axes than those about which the single rotating forces attempt to rotate the eye alone. The last example shows the opposite, that one can think of any rotation of the eye as consisting of two simultaneous rotations put together, where one occurs about an axis which is perpendicular to the line of sight and to the current direction of movement and the other occurs about the line of sight itself. It does not matter where the moment of rotation and the axes lie about which the movement really occurs. Such an analysis of the rotations is no longer possible if the real rotation already occurs about axes which are perpendicular to the line of sight, because then the rotation about the line of sight is zero. It is also impossible when the true rotation occurs about the line of sight itself. Of course, every real rotation of the eyes can also be thought of as analyzed into simultaneous rotations about any other axes, and this example was chosen only because of other considerations below.

It is known that straight line movements of a body follow the same rules as the forces which elicit these movements. If point *a* (Figure 10) moves first to *c* and then from *c* to *b,* or first to *d* and then from *d* to *b,* and I observe the two described paths as sides of a parallelogram, then the diagonal *ab* describes the direction and length of the path on which the point *a* could be moved directly to *b.* I can therefore substitute this simple movement for the double movement of the point without changing the end result. It is different with two successive rotations. One might want to put the true rotation together in the same way as the moments of rotation, that is, to extend the half axes of the two rotations from the point of rotation so that the sizes (angles) of the two rotations were proportional, to consider these extended portions as sides of a parallelogram, and to construct its diagonal. But this process would in no way give the half axes and sizes of the simple rotations through which the body to be considered came into this position after the accomplishment of the two rotations.

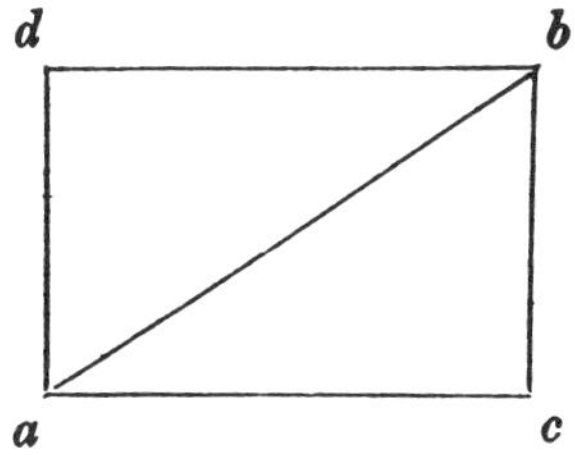

Fig. 10.

To make this clear the beginner should insert three pins *v*, *h*, and *g* through a ball at right angles to one another so that their crossing point represents the rotation point of the eye. Needle *v* is oriented vertically while the other two, *h* and *g*, are horizontal. One of these, *g*, can be labeled as the representation of the line of sight. Now one can rotate the ball 90° about the vertical needle as an axis so the line of sight *g* and the third needle *h* are displaced about 90°. Both, however, remain horizontal during and after the rotation. Then rotate the ball in another way, specifically about the needle *h*, again through 90°; this needle will remain horizontal, *v* will move away from the vertical position to a horizontal one and *g* out of the horizontal into the vertical.

Now bring the needles to their original position again and make the same rotation in the reverse order, that is, rotate first about the horizontal needle *h* through 90° so that the line of sight *g* moves out of the horizontal position into the vertical, but the needle *v* moves out of the vertical into a horizontal position. Now rotate the ball about the latter needle *v* through 90°; it remains horizontal, the line of sight *g* will move from vertical to horizontal and the needle *h* will move from the horizontal to the vertical orientation.

Thus we have rotated axes *v* and *h* through 90° both times, but the end result the first time was that the line of sight was finally vertical while the second time it finally had a horizontal position, and correspondingly the final positions of the needles *v* and *h* were different in both cases.

Thus the fact that the ball comes to a completely different position according to whether one or the other of the two rotations occurs first makes it clear that two rotations cannot be combined in the same way as the moments of rotation. Now take equal distances along the two axes h and v each according to the half axes describing the direction of rotation, consider these as sides of a quadrilateral, and construct the diagonal between them. One will not be able to bring the ball into one of the two positions which we have found as end results of the two rotations by rotating about axes on this diagonal (which makes an angle of 45° with h and v).

The dependence of the end result on the sequence of the two rotations, which came to light so clearly because of the large extent of the rotations in the example, occurs to a proportionately smaller degree with smaller rotations and disappears only when the two rotations are infinitely small. Thus, only infinitely small rotations can be combined with the same rules as the moments of rotation. This corresponds to cutting pieces from the half axes which are proportional to the sizes of rotation, and considering these pieces as sides of a parallelogram whose diagonal gives the half axis and the size of the corresponding single infinitely small rotation through which the ball can be brought into the same position as through the *two* successive infinitely small rotations. If one wants to substitute a single rotation for many rotations of finite size, so that the end position of the ball is the same in both cases, the necessary axis is easy to find if one knows the ball's beginning position L and its end position L'. Both positions are determined if the locations of two diameters (for instance, g and v) are given before and after the rotation. One now constructs a plane E through the bisecting line of the angle which the beginning position of one diameter (g) makes with its end position and perpendicular to the plane of this angle, and analogously bisects the angle which the beginning position of the other diameter (v) makes with its end position with a plane E' perpendicular to the plane of this angle. The diameter in which these two planes E and E' intersect is then the desired fixed axis about which one can rotate the ball directly from the given beginning position L into the given end position L'.

14. *The Law of Equal Retinal Position with Equal Fixation Position*

From the rule of eye movement described above it follows that every specific position of the fixation point in bifixation space corresponds to a quite specific state of contraction of specific eye muscle groups, which always occurs when the fixation of the double eye comes to lie on the same point of the fixation space. So, if the gaze rests on a point *A* to the right and above in the far distance, for instance, a given shortening of the raisers and right-turners will be necessary to hold fixation there. This shortening will always occur to exactly the same degree whenever fixation returns to point *A* with unchanged head position after any deviation. At the same time, all other eye muscles will always show the same conditions of passive tension as long as their elastic forces are not somehow changed. Thus all other forces working on the eyeball will also be the same and will work in the same directions. It follows that not only the line of sight but also every other point of the eyeball and the retina (which is of special interest to us here) will always have the same position. Briefly, *the cyclorotary orientation of the eyes will be a single valued function of the fixation position.* If we create a lasting afterimage on a given retinal meridian of one eye with a small colored strip of paper and turn our fixation to any object, with the afterimage in the eye, then the afterimage will always cover exactly the same parts of the object whenever we bring fixation to the same point on the object after any deviations. Every individual point of the object will be imaged on the same point of the retina if neither the head nor the object is moved. In the following paragraphs the correctness of this statement will be illustrated with numerous experiments.

With the same position of the line of sight of an eye relative to the head, the point of sight can have various positions because the line of sight of the other eye can intersect that of the first at various points. Now I have shown above that when the left line of sight is fixed straight ahead, for instance, and the right one moves along the left one, that is if the point of sight comes closer from the distance, then not only the moved right eye but also the left experiences a change in innervation corresponding to this nearing. In spite of the always-constant position of the left line of sight, the tension of the single muscles of the left eye can thus be significantly different, as is usually revealed through a changed orientation of the eyeball. As will be shown later, a small involuntary rolling of eye about the line of sight occurs if one holds the latter fixed but brings the fixated point nearer or further away along the line of sight such that the other line of sight changes its position.

The orientation of the eye therefore depends not only on the position of its line of sight in visual space, as previously assumed (Donders), but also on the position of the line of sight of the other eye.

As already indicated, our will directs itself only to changing the position of the point of sight or maintaining it at a given location. The cyclorotary position which the retina assumes is dependent in a purely mechanical way on the tension of the muscles which occurs for the purpose of movement or of maintaining the point of sight. It is, therefore, only partially and not completely dominated by the will. Just as we indirectly change our heartbeat by voluntarily holding the breath, although it is impossible to change this directly with an impulse of the will, so we can also change cyclorotary position by moving the point of sight. Specifically, as already said, with a fixed line of sight of one eye we can roll that eye slightly about the line of sight although we are not accustomed to initiate such a rolling through a direct impulse of will. For vision under normal conditions, the voluntary rolling of the eye about its line of sight would generally have no purpose, though it would indeed be desirable in specific pathological cases and under artificially changed conditions in the interest of clear vision; nonetheless, it is not possible in either case for the seeing person.

One can, for instance, cut the two halves of an ordinary stereoscopic picture apart and first place the pictures in the stereoscope in the ordinary way, obtain the stereoscopic fused image, fix one point of the same firmly in the eye, and then rotate one half-picture slowly about the fixated point. As soon as this rotation exceeds a certain fairly small angle, the fused image breaks up and one sees two pictures through one another, where one appears rotated against the other. Thus only the fixated points will be seen single and all others doubled. This would not occur if we were able in the interest of clear vision to roll one eye about the line of sight to the same extent to which the image which it sees is rotated, or to roll both eyes each about half of the angle. In either case simple and meaningful vision would again become possible.

There is not a single well-investigated case where someone has been able to roll the eyes about the line of sight with unchanged position of the point of sight; a contrary declaration by Helmholtz will be discussed below. This should not imply that some methods may not indeed be found through which one can achieve these movements so to say in an unnatural way. Further, just as there are men who once accidentally have found the innervation for one movement which is not possible for anyone else, so it would also be conceivable that someone might by chance find the innervation necessary for rolling the eyes about the line of sight. I have shown examples myself above which prove that it is not only simple spatial conceptions through which we can induce innervation of the eye muscles. The influence of affect on eye movement delivers enough examples of this. Many people are able to make quite exceptional artificial movements with their muscles. It is known that many can wiggle their ears; I myself know someone who can fold the free edge of his tongue in folds like a ruffle, and there are many similar curiosities. Eye rolling might thus be possible in this way, although until now nothing certain is known about it. A rolling of the eyes brought about in this way would of course be without special meaning for the theory of eye movements in the interest of vision. But if true cases of small voluntary rolling of the eyes in the interest of meaningful vision are proved, the laws described in the above paragraphs would be just as little disturbed as the rule of equal innervation of both eyes is made invalid by the possibility of weak one-sided raising or lowering of an eye under special circumstances.

Moreover, it has been mentioned that the rule of equal retinal position with equal fixation position suffers small exceptions if the elasticity or power of a specific muscle is changed by strenuous use. Thus, one finds temporarily that if one goes from one fixation position to another, in the first moment the position of the retinas does not exactly correspond to the fixation position. But the normal orientation is soon restored. These phenomena, already noted by Helmholtz, I can completely confirm.

Though it had been widely accepted earlier that the eye could execute a rolling about a fixed site, Donders showed that retinal position is always the same with equal position of the line of sight. Through numerous experiments this rule has been shown to be very nearly correct for distant fixation points, though it is no longer applicable as soon as the lines of sight converge, as will be thoroughly demonstrated below.

The law formulated by Donders and which is strictly correct for parallel positions leads immediately to the consequence that a voluntary rolling of the eye about the line of sight is impossible. This conclusion, moreover, finds extensive confirmation in stereoscopic experiments. For instance, if one sets up two straight lines tilted toward one another, each on one side of a vertical plane parallel to the lines of sight so that only one line is visible to each eye, then with *steady fixation* one is not able to fuse the two lines into a single image as long as their angle of inclination exceeds a certain amount. And if the lines are fine this angle of inclination is very small for those who are practiced in steady fixation and indirect vision. When one fixates their middle point the lines appear as two lines intersecting with a small angle at the fixation point. It is apparent that the fusing of the lines would immediately be possible if the eyes could execute a small rolling about the line of sight so that the retinal images of the two lines came to lie on identical meridians. Now, since other eye movements are known to be executed in the service of fused vision it would be remarkable that rolling about the line of sight, if it could be executed voluntarily, did not occur in this case. One also notes that as long as the paper and the head remain steady there is no change at all in the apparent angle of inclination of the two intersection lines, from which it follows that the two eyes make no effort to the purpose of fused vision in spite of the different positions of the retinal images.

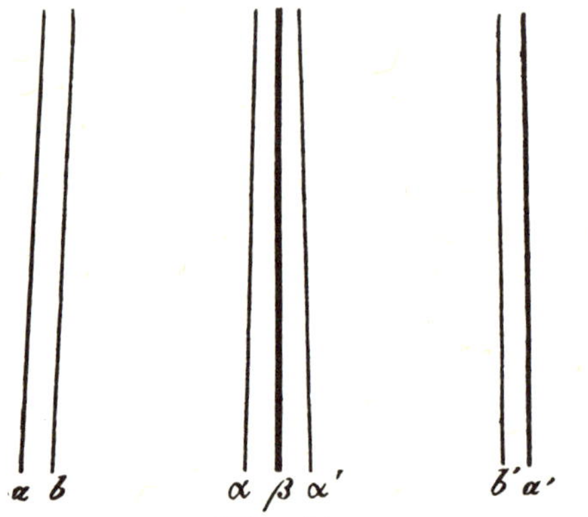

Fig. 11.

If the two lines have a position differentiated only enough that they can still be fused into a single image with steady fixation, and if one wants to judge this fact without relationship to other further stereoscopic experiences, then one can come to the idea that the fusion of the two lines was brought about because the two lines which originally laid on different retinal meridians were transferred to identical meridians by rolling of the eyes. But this assumption is easy to disprove. Specifically, if one offers to each eye two parallel lines instead of one, having the same orientations as the single lines before, and binocularly fuses the two inner lines b and b' (Figure 11), then one sees three lines a, B, and a', of which the middle one B represents the fused image of the two inner lines, while the line a' appearing to the right is seen only by the right eye and the line a is seen only by the left. But these two monocularly seen lines do not appear parallel, as they would have to if the two retinal images of the inner lines were positioned on identical meridians. They appear divergent, expressing the difference of the retinal lines on which they are imaged. If one has further achieved a fused image from two lines which create only slightly different retinal images, the fused image dissipates at once into two apparently divergent lines if one slightly increases or decreases the convergent angle of the lines of sight. This also could not occur if the eyes had undergone a rolling, for according to other observations it cannot be assumed that the eyes could compensate so quickly with opposed rolling. If one draws the two lines on two separate papers and moves them quickly apart or together after one has achieved the fused image, the line which before appeared single dissociates into two divergent ones. This proves conclusively that the eyes have not rolled, for otherwise the lines would have to appear as a parallel pair of lines in the moment of the dissociation of the fused image. These facts, which should indeed be familiar to everyone who has occupied himself with stereoscopic experiments, confirm adequately the rule of always-equal position of the retina with equal position of the point of sight and forbid the assumption of a voluntary rolling of the eye about the line of sight. This is even more true because such a rolling has no *a priori* probability for other reasons.

On the basis of new observations Helmholtz has recently asserted that even the rolling of the eyes about the line of sight "is subject to the will and can be called forth whenever it is necessary for the only possible intention of will which can be established for eye movement, namely fused and clear vision." Although I believed that through my previous experiments I had already adequately convinced myself that this is not true, I have indeed undertaken further experimental testing of this matter. This has led to a thorough confirmation of the previous results. At the same time, it became clear that Helmholtz arrived at his conclusion only because the path of the light rays in the optical apparatus which he used was not adequately controlled.

Helmholtz set before himself the task of creating apparent cyclorotation of the entire field of vision of one eye with optical methods, while for the other eye the apparent position of the field of vision remained unchanged. He then investigated whether the general double vision thus created could again be corrected by a rolling of the eyes, and he believed that he found this to be the case.

Because it is irrelevant for the experiment whether one creates the necessary retinal images with external objects themselves or with a good photograph of them, the Helmholtz apparatus need not be used. The experiment can be arranged in any good stereoscope if one separates the two single images from one another and fastens small knobs on them so that both images can be rotated about corresponding points. It is then apparent that without any further optical apparatus the fields of sight of the two eyes can be rotated at will against one another. If one arranges the experiments in this way it is easy to convince oneself that everything behaves exactly as I have described it above in the experiment with the two vertical lines, with the single difference that the fusion of the two images occurs relatively more easily because linear and air perspective, etc., aid it. If one has once fused the two images which are rotated against one another and moves them slightly together or apart while at the same time holding a prominent vertical contour of the image in the eye, one sees (or at least can immediately make noticeable by weak shaking) that the double contour into which the previously fused image thereby decays always has the divergence that one noted at the beginning of the experiment. Here it is completely irrelevant how long one has been occupied with the images; in spite of long duration of the experiment, no compensatory rolling of the eyes occurs. Another modification of the experiment consists of positioning the pictures at the beginning such that they image identically on the retinas and then, while constantly viewing the fused image, slowly introducing a rotation of one or both images about corresponding points. Of course, the stereoscopic effect is somewhat changed with this according to the direction of the rotation. When the images are rotated so far that one has difficulty in seeing them fused, or if the splitting into two intersecting images has just occurred, one ends the rotation and attempts as long as possible to eliminate the many double images in such contrasting pictures through a small rolling. But not a trace of this ever occurs. I will further note that Dr. Becker, a well known and practiced observer in binocular vision experiments, arranged the experiment with the same negative results.

I have noted that Helmholtz did not use the simple apparatus just discussed for his experiments, but used a complicated one which, however, does not exactly fulfill the requirements of the experiments. One looks at a distant object through an equal-sided right-angle prism whose edges are perpendicular to the direction of the line of sight while the hypotenuse surface is parallel to it (see

Figure 12). Because of the total reflection of the light rays on the latter surface, one then sees the objects behind the prism as distorted. The inversion of the image depends upon the position of the prism. Right and left are exchanged if the hypotenuse surface is vertical, while up and down are exchanged if it is horizontal. The only points which do not change their position have a particular central position; in the first case these are the fixation point and the points which appear vertically over or under it, and in the second case the fixation point along with the points which appear to the left and right at the same height. Rotation of this prism about the line of sight as an axis then elicits an apparent rotation about the fixated point, whose angle is twice as large as the angle of rotation of the prism. For example, with a 45° tilt of the hypotenuse surface from the horizontal, a vertical line will seem horizontal and a horizontal vertical. One now holds a second identical prism in front of or behind the first so that the hypotenuse surfaces and the edges of both prisms are parallel. The inversion of the field of sight is now doubled, i.e., it appears in the natural position again. One then rotates one prism about the line of sight as an axis. Obviously, the field of vision must then experience an apparent rotation, and again about twice the angle of the true rotation of the prism, except that one now has the advantage that this rotation occurs in isolation, without the former simultaneous inversion of right and left or up and down when only one prism was used. (This is a description of the modern "Dove prism." – B.B.)

With this double prism one has a means of rotating the entire visual space of one eye about the line of sight as an axis and thereby reaching the analog of rotating one of the two stereoscopic pictures about the line of sight. The corresponding results are exactly the same as those of the experiments with stereoscopic pictures discussed above. If one rotates one prism slightly one sees singly as before, except that for well-practiced observers a small change of the position of external objects sometimes appears in the depth dimension. For instance, vertical objects no longer appear vertical but somewhat angled forward or backward just as the rules of binocular depth perception require. These changes in apparent position are indeed partly corrected for well known objects of vision by our knowledge of their true position. But a compensatory rolling of the eyes about the line of sight never occurs in spite of the rotation of one retinal image.

If Helmholtz had arranged the prisms in the described way he would not have come to the conclusion that the eyes execute compensatory rolling movements. But he proceeded in another way; namely, he rotated one prism against the other after he had placed the two short-sided surfaces against one another. Rotation occurred about an axis perpendicular to one of these surfaces, that is, about an axis which enclosed an angle of 45° between the hypotenuse surfaces and the line of sight, but was not parallel to the line of sight as the conditions of the experiment require. With the prisms arranged in this way, he glued the short surfaces to one another. With such an arrangement the apparent rotation of the field of vision occurs not about the line of sight, that is not about the fixated point, but about one which is more or less eccentric in the field of vision. The result is that the middle part of the field of vision is displaced in an arc upward or downward and simultaneously right or left. Thus double images arise, either symmetrical or unsymmetrical, at various heights and these rotate against one another. The double images usually disappear because one eye begins to squint inward or outward and at the same time upward or downward in order to bring the double images into fusion. As soon as the vertical or lateral deviation of the two images is compensated by this squint, one sees single images again, provided that the rotation of the two images against one another is not so great that a stereoscopic fusion is impossible.

Helmholtz incorrectly interpreted the appearance of double images solely as a result of the rotation of the retinal images, neglecting their lateral and vertical distortion. He took the fusion which occurred after a while to be the result of a compensatory rolling of the eyes about the line of sight, though they are only the result of a compensatory squint of one eye. Helmholtz's other results on the apparent locations of the double images in this experiment and the positions of afterimages which he could elicit in the eye equipped with a prism are invalid because he did not take account of the deviation of the line of sight of the eye, which must be abnormally innervated for the purpose of focusing the line of sight. Thus the orientation of the retina can also be different than if the eye were not equipped with a prism.

As they stand these experiments prove nothing about the existence of a voluntary rolling of the eye about the line of sight. Because I myself could not find such a rolling in performing this experiment (as expressed in the above exposition), and because Dr. Becker has been equally unsuccessful with the experiments with stereoscopic images described above (which have exactly the same demonstrative power), I judge the hypothesis of voluntary eye rolling as unproved for the present. As I have said above, I will not contest their possibility.

For those who want to repeat this experiment I still want to describe the way I have arranged the prisms. They are inserted in two short wooden cylinders, and these cylinders are inserted in the two open ends of a short brass tube in which they can rotate. The opposing positions of the prisms are such that the ray of light which coincides with the axis of the apparatus before its entrance again coincides with this axis after its exit, with any desired rotation of the two prisms relative to one another. Figure 12 shows the path of this ray through the prisms, where both hypotenuse surfaces lie parallel. The prisms are brought as close as possible to one another so that an adequate rotation is just possible. The tube with the prisms must be firmly fixed and may not be held with the hand, and in addition, if one wants to do experiments with afterimages, the head must also be fixed if other similar experiments are to be convincing. But because the experiment with the prisms cannot after all prove anything more than the experiment with the two images which are rotatable with respect to one another and binocularly fusible, the latter is more practical.

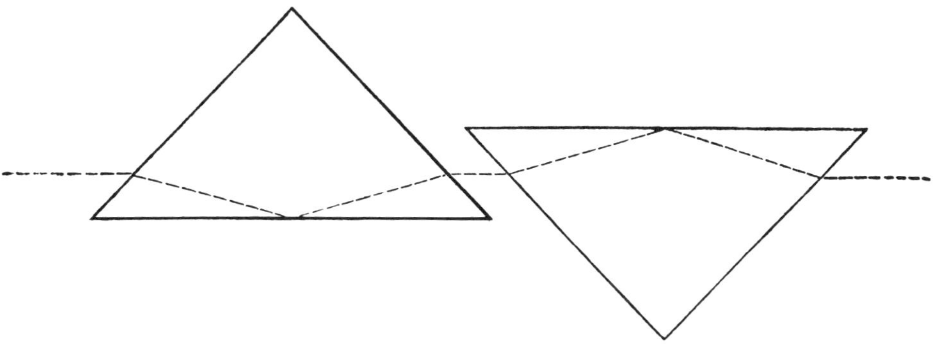

Fig. 12.

15. *The Law of Orientation with Parallel Lines of Sight*

As discussed in chapter 13, the line of sight can move with or without simultaneous rotation. So that the latter movements can be differentiated in terminology from the other rotations of the eye I will give them the special name of *rolling* (cyclorotation in modern terminology – B.B.). This rolling has been previously termed circular rotation (Raddrehung), but because this word is often used in a quite different sense in the opthalmological literature it appears appropriate to me to avoid it here in the interest of clarity.

If the line of sight is to move without a simultaneous rolling of the eyes, then the axis of rotation must remain perpendicular to the path of the rotation of the line of sight at every moment, i.e., it must always make a right angle with the line of sight. The line of sight thus describes a plane in this special case and the axis of rotation must be perpendicular to this plane and always the same, that is, it must be a *fixed axis.* On the other hand, if the line of sight moves with a simultaneous rolling of the eyes the momentary axis of rotation will describe any other desired angle with the line of sight, and if the line of sight thus describes a plane, then the rotation will occur not about a fixed axis but about *momentary axes.* Movements of the line of sight with which the eye is simultaneously rolled, that is, eye movements which can be thought of as combined from a movement of the line of sight on one hand and a rolling of the eyes on the other in the manner of chapter 13 occur frequently in reality.

With distance vision there is a certain position of the line of sight (relative to the head), the so-called *primary position,* from which the *line of sight can describe a path in any direction, or fixation can follow any straight line, without the eye experiencing any rotation about the line of sight,* that is, a position from which *the eye can be rotated in all directions about a fixed axis perpendicular to the line of sight.* This rule was first proposed by Listing and is named *Listing's Law* after him. As already shown by Listing and confirmed by Helmholtz, the primary position specified above appears not to deviate very much from the position which a free erect holding of the head requires in normal-sighted people, with both lines of sight horizontal and positioned parallel straight ahead.

If one positions himself in a large room at the middle of one wall, with the back and the back of the head leaned against the wall, and fixates a point *P* which is on the opposite wall at the same height as the eyes and directly in front of them, then both eyes will be nearly in the primary position. (This will not usually be exactly the case because the point of sight does not lie far enough away that the lines of sight may be assumed to be parallel or because one does not find the exactly correct position of the head. But I will assume that the eyes are fortuitously exactly in the primary position. I will reserve for the following paragraphs a description of more exact methods with which one can find the primary position and can prove Listing's Law more exactly.) On the wall four threads (in a color contrasting with that of the wall) are strung so that they all intersect at the point of sight *P*, one horizontal, one vertical, and the other two each at 45° to the first two. A long thin strip of firm cardboard, covered on one side with a paper whose color contrasts well with that of the wall, is fixed to the point *P* with a nail at its middle point so that it can be rotated with some friction about the nail as an axis. The color of the cardboard strip can be red if the wall is green, or green if the latter is red, blue if it is yellow, or of any other intensive color if the wall is white. The colored strip should now be so positioned that it comes to lie at the position of one of the four threads, that is, exactly under one of them. One should now fixate the middle point of the strip (the point *P*) in order to create an afterimage of the strip. Then let fixation move along the thread on which the colored strip lies. Note that the afterimage of the strip appears to lie on the thread for its entire length and that both long sides lie parallel to the thread. One now rotates the strip to the direction of another thread, creates another afterimage and glances along the thread; the afterimage always appears on the thread. In this manner one can repeat the experiment on each of the four threads in different position, or further on any other straight line intersecting the point *P*; the long side of the afterimage always remains parallel to the line followed by the fixation if the colored strip was exactly on this line beforehand.

During the fixation of the point *P*, one can imagine a plane *E* which intersects both the line of sight and the straight line or string coinciding with the strip which elicits afterimages. This plane intersects the retina in the meridian *M* where the string *S* and the colored strip are imaged. If the line of sight then moves along the string *S* while remaining in the plane *E* it is apparent that the retinal image of the string must always remain in the plane *E* and, if no rolling of the eyes about the line of sight occurs, it must also remain on the meridian *M*. But the afterimage also lies on this meridian; with this movement is always appears to lie on the string *S* and appears to move only in the direction of the string. Had a rolling of the eyes occurred during this movement of the line of sight, the meridian *M* (and with it the superimposed afterimage from the plane *E*) would be rotated, which means that the afterimage of the string *S* would be more or less tilted on the retina. Correspondingly it would appear on the wall at an oblique angle to the string *S*.

If the cardboard strip lies perpendicular to one of the strings while the eye fixates it in the primary position, and one then lets his fixation run along this string, then the afterimage appears to be always perpendicular to this string, though it would appear to be tilted with respect to the string if a rolling of the eyes had taken place during the movement.

One can imagine all possible planes which intersect the line of sight when it is in the primary position. These are called *the primary meridian planes* and they describe the sum of the paths which the line of sight can assume without the occurrence of a rolling of the eyes about the line of sight. Further, imagine all possible diameters perpendicular to the line of sight and through the point of rotation of the eye in primary position. These represent the axes about which the eye can be rotated away from the primary position. The sum of these primary axes constructs a plane which lies perpendicular to the line of sight and which can be called the *plane of primary axes.*

But now it can be shown that the line of sight can be brought from a given position to any other possible position by rotation about fixed axes perpendicular to the line of sight. This does not apply analogously from the other positions of the line of sight, given that the entire eye always has the same position when the line of sight returns to the same place. Rather, Listing's Law has a theoretically necessary corollary that *if the line of sight describes a path not from the primary position but from any other position, the rotation cannot occur about fixed axes perpendicular to the line of sight, that is, it cannot occur without a simultaneous rolling of the eyes except in the single case that the plane in which the line of sight moves simultaneously intersects the primary position itself,* and is therefore one of the primary meridian planes defined above.

This can easily be shown experimentally if one repeats the experiment just discussed after tilting the head forward or back, to the right, to the left, or in some other way. If one again fixates the point *P,* the lines of sight are then indeed in the same position relative to the observation wall as they were with an upright head. But they now lie differently relative to the latter and are therefore no longer in their primary position, but in another so-called *secondary position,* which is the name of every position which is not the primary position. If one again elicits an afterimage under such conditions and lets his fixation move along the string on which the colored stripe lies, one notices that the afterimage does not remain lying on the string but is rotated away from it and intersects it at an oblique angle. The eye has rotated about the line of sight during this movement in the same direction in which the afterimage rotates away from the string. For instance, if one had nodded the head forward and now looked along the horizontal string, then the originally horizontal afterimage would rotate more and more away from the direction of the stripe as the fixation deviated further to the right or left. On the other hand, if one now experiments with the vertical string with the same head position and with a vertical afterimage, the afterimage remains on the vertical strings if one looks up or down along the string. In the latter case, the line of sight moves specifically in a plane which also contains the primary position, namely in the primary vertical meridian plane. If one makes any movement other than a vertical one with this head position, a small deviation of the afterimage from the string will reveal a rolling of the eyes.

Until now we have experimented only with afterimages which, with the eyes in primary position, lay along or perpendicular to the line along which the gaze subsequently moved. It is very important to become familiar with the apparent position of the afterimage under other conditions as well.

Assume that an eye finds itself in the primary position again, with its line of sight horizontal and oriented toward the point *P* on a wall vertical to the line of sight. If a colored strip of paper is applied vertically on the wall through this point, it will be imaged on the vertical retinal meridian *V* and will elicit an afterimage on that meridian with steady fixation of the point *P*. Divide the entire wall into squares with vertical and horizontal lines. If the line of sight is now displaced upward or downward or horizontally to the left or right with unchanged head position, then the afterimage on the wall will always appear vertical. But as soon as fixation moves upward or downward in an oblique direction, the afterimage will appear tilted on the wall. Analogous results are obtained if the colored strip which elicits the afterimage is not vertical but horizontal through the point *P*. Or if one places a horizontal and a vertical stripe simultaneously through the point *P*, that is, a colored right-angled cross, then the afterimage of the cross will be right-angled with one arm appearing horizontal and the other vertical as long as fixation is directed toward a horizontal or vertical line on the wall through the point *P*. The cross will, on the other hand, appear non-rectangular and its arms will be neither horizontal nor vertical if the point of sight deviates significantly in any way from the two lines. Figure 13 shows the wall with the horizontal and vertical lines, while the black cross in the middle represents the colored cross whose fixation elicits the afterimage. The other crosses represent the afterimage as it appears on the wall with various positions of the point of sight.

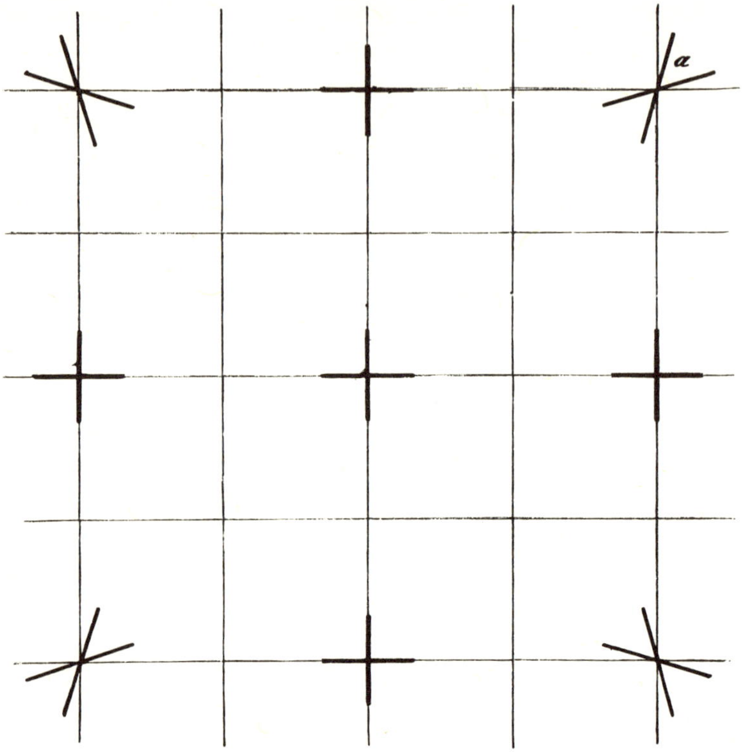

Fig. 13.

This change in position of the two arms of the cross in the afterimage and the apparent distortion of its form occurs because the vertically right-angled cross lines on the wall are not imaged at right angles on the retina, but have an oblique intersection as soon as the line of sight is placed obliquely to the wall in the above manner. At point *a* in figure 13, for instance, a horizontal and a vertical line intersect at right angles on the wall; if the line of sight is now placed on this point, the two lines project on the retina in the same way as the lines *hh* and *vv* in figure 14A, while the afterimage of the colored cross on the retina of course remains right-angled as before, as the black cross in the same figure shows. But now because we see the intersecting lines on the wall as right-angled in spite of their oblique-angled retinal image (for reasons which will be discussed below), that is, we see the four angles *vah* (figure 14A) all as right angles, we must in like manner see the retinal right angle of the afterimage as oblique, and the afterimage therefore appears to us as in figure 14B. The cause of this distortion of the afterimage is therefore solely the way in which we arrange the afterimage, for we perceive the vertical and horizontal lines on the wall to be vertical and horizontal as before in spite of the oblique-angled retinal image.

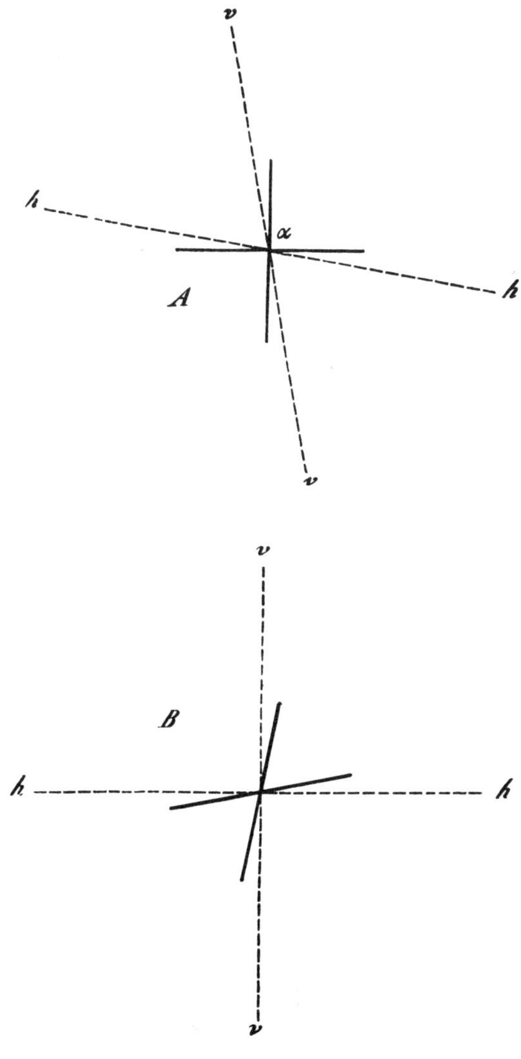

Fig. 14.

Now if we had laid only one vertical colored strip on the wall through the primary point *P*, obtained an afterimage from it, and then moved fixation in a straight line diagonally above and to the right to point *a* in figure 13, then the afterimage during this movement would have changed its apparent position and turned its upper end to the right. As in fact has often happened, this could lead to the erroneous conclusion that the eye had experienced a rolling about the line of sight during the movement, though the true origin of the apparent rotation of the afterimage is solely that the vertical lines on the wall are no longer imaged in the primary position vertical meridian or one parallel to it. Instead their images on the retina seem to rotate because of changed projection relationships during the movement. Had the colored strip been horizontal during the primary fixation of the point *P* and had the line of sight then traveled directly from *P* to *a*, then the afterimage of the strip with this movement would also have experienced an apparent rotation, but in the direction opposite from the previous vertical strip: the left end of the afterimage would tip downward. This dependence of the direction of the apparent rotation of the afterimage on its original position already proves that a rolling of the eye about the line of sight cannot be the origin of this phenomenon. Had the colored strip (and with it also its afterimage) been in the primary position at the orientation of the line connecting points *P* and *a*, or perpendicular to it, then as was shown above, the afterimage would show no apparent rotation with direct transfer of fixation from *P* to *a*.

Thus if one wants to gain information about the orientation of the retina from the apparent rotation of the afterimage, one must pay attention to how and to what extent the altered form and position of the retinal image depends on the external objects on which the afterimage appears, and with whose lines and contours the position of the afterimage will be compared.

If one wants to determine with an afterimage whether and how a rolling of the eyes occurs while fixation moves at will along a straight line in space, it is most effective to orient the afterimage-eliciting stripe with its length on the line itself. If one moves fixation along this line and the afterimage does not remain on it but rotates away from it, then a rolling of the eyes has certainly occurred, specifically in the same direction in which the afterimage appeared to rotate, though not about the same angle. For the angle of the apparent rotation of the afterimage is not dependent solely on the rolling of the eyes but can also appear larger or smaller depending upon the orientation of the surface on which the afterimage appears.

Figure 15 shows the apparent position which an originally vertical afterimage assumes on a vertical plane, given that the line of sight in the primary position intersects the point *P* perpendicularly. Further, the afterimage-eliciting strip goes vertically through the point *P*, the head is held fixed in spite of the moving of the eyes, and *ab* is the direct separation between the rotation point of the eye and the vertical plane. If one thinks of this distance and the figure

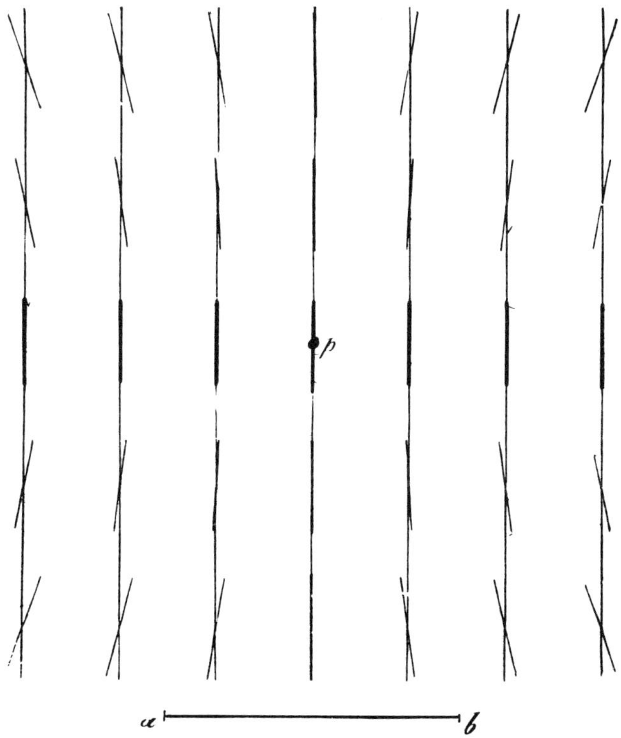

Fig. 15.

expanded to the same degree, then the figure applies for any given distance of the eye from the vertical plane. The retina has the same position in the orbit whenever the line of sight in far vision comes again to the same place, so that the originally vertical afterimage always returns to the same apparent position when fixation falls again on the same point (given an unchanged position of the head and the observation plane). At the same time figure 15 also gives a picture of the rotation which the afterimage experiences while fixation moves in any direction over the plane. As already noted, these rotations are indeed a pure expression of the rolling of the eyes only if the path of eye movement is vertical or horizontal.

The afterimage rotates clockwise, if fixation rises from right below to right above, as the figure shows. If fixation moves downward on the same line, then the rotation is the opposite, and if it rises from left below to left above, then the afterimage rotates its upper end to the left. With lowering of fixation from left above to left below, it rotates to the right. The eye is now rolled about the line of sight in the same way as the afterimage in the movements just described. The figure also shows that the rotation of the afterimage and the corresponding rolling of the eyes is stronger the further the vertical fixation line deviates from the vertical through the point *P*. As already shown, no rotation occurs with movement of gaze along the latter.

If we let fixation run along not a vertical path but an otherwise-oriented straight path on the vertical plane (the plane of figure 15 – B.B.), then we see that rotations of the afterimage also occur, as the figure shows. But these are partly or entirely the result of the changed projection and give us no direct information about how and in which way the rolling of the eyes has occurred. If one wants to know whether and in which way a rolling of the eyes occurs in such cases, one can think of figure 15 as rotated about its middle point *P* far enough that the originally vertical lines of the figure lie parallel to the lines along which fixation is to move. The afterimage position illustrated in the figure then gives the direction of the rolling. If the line through which fixation is to move is tilted 45° from the horizontal, then one must rotate the figure 45° about its middle point. If fixation then moves along the given line, for instance from the lower left to above right, and if this line runs below the primary position of the line of sight, then the rotation of the afterimage (and the rolling of the eye) will occur with the upper part to the right, and will be larger the further the line deviates from the middle point *P* of the field of fixation. If figure 15 is rotated far enough that the long strips lie horizontal, then it shows the rotation which a horizontal afterimage experiences, and the corresponding rolling of the eyes which occurs when one moves fixation along one of the horizontal lines, etc.

Thus, assuming that fixation moves over distant objects, the eye experiences no rolling about the line of sight during movements which occur in a plane which simultaneously contains the primary position, that is in a primary meridian plane. A constant rolling of the eyes occurs if the line of sight describes some other plane or path. But these rollings are very small, so small that they practically never come into consideration as long as fixation remains in smaller fixation space, that is, remains in the space which it never leaves in ordinary vision. These rollings would be disturbing even in smaller fixation space if a very exact orientation about the directions of lines were necessary. But in such cases we take care to orient to the investigated line so that it comes to lie in a meridian plane of the primary position.

What I have identified above as rolling is usually called *circular rotation* (Raddrehung), or *rotation projected on the line of sight.* From Listing's Law, which I will show to apply only for the eye looking in the distance, it follows that *if the line of sight lies in the upper right or lower left quadrants of fixation space, the primary vertical meridian* (but note, not the vertical dividing line) *deviates with its upper end to the left from the position vertical to the plane of fixation, and the primary horizontal meridian is rotated with its left end below the plane of fixation. The opposite is the case if the line of sight finds itself in the other two quadrants.* Thus, fixation space is thought of as divided by a horizontal and a vertical plane which contain the horizontal line coinciding with the line of sight in the primary position. Helmholtz has calculated the angle of this meridional deviation for the various positions of the line of sight under the assumption of the absolute applicability of Listing's Law and summarized them in the following table. The deviation of the plane of fixation from the primary position is labeled "raising" in the table, so that one can think of sinking as negative raising. The sideward deviation from the medial direction which the line of sight assumes in any plane of fixation is labeled sideward turning.

Though table 1 applies for all four quarters of fixation space, one must consider that in the upper right and lower left quarters the deviation of the primary meridian from the position vertical to the fixation plane is the opposite from that which occurs in the upper left and lower right quarters.

Some geometric inferences from Listing's Law. Assume that the line of sight of the eye can be brought from a given (primary) loca-

Table 1

Raising Angle

Sideward Deviation	5°	10°	15°	20°	25°	30°	35°	40°
5°	0° 13′	0° 26′	0° 40′	0° 53′	1° 7′	1° 20′	1° 35′	1° 49′
10°	0° 26′	0° 53′	1° 19′	1° 46′	2° 13′	2° 41′	3° 10′	3° 39′
15°	0° 40′	1° 19′	1° 59′	2° 40′	3° 21′	4° 2′	4° 45′	5° 29′
20°	0° 53′	1° 46′	2° 40′	3° 34′	4° 29′	5° 25′	6° 22′	7° 21′
25°	1° 7′	2° 13′	3° 21′	4° 29′	5° 38′	6° 48′	8° 0′	9° 14′
30°	1° 21′	2° 41′	4° 2′	5° 25′	6° 48′	8° 13′	9° 39′	11° 8′
35°	1° 35′	3° 10′	4° 45′	6° 22′	8° 0′	9° 39′	11° 21′	13° 6′
40°	1° 49′	3° 39′	5° 29′	7° 21′	9° 14′	11° 8′	13° 6′	15° 5′

tion into any other (secondary) location by rotating the eye about a fixed axis at right angles to the line of sight, and further, that every given position of the line of sight is inflexibly related to a given position of the eye. Several further noteworthy conclusions then follow:

(1) In the primary position all axes about which the eye can begin a rotation lie in one plane. This applies also from every secondary position except that in the latter case the plane of the axes has another position relative to the line of sight.

(2) With every eye movement the plane of the axes changes its position as much in the eye as in the head, that is, both with respect to a coordinate system fixed with respect to the eye and moving with it and with respect to a coordinate system fixed with respect to the head. The plane of the axes does not have the same position for any two eye positions.

(3) The plane of the axes moves along the same axes as the eye rotation, and specifically *in the eye* in the opposite direction (about the opposite half axes) as the eye itself. But it moves in the same direction *in the head* (with the same half axes) as the eye, though in both cases with only half the angular speed.

(4) The eye can be moved from any secondary position to any other secondary position by rotation about a fixed axis, where it again moves through secondary positions and the line of sight generally describes a conic surface. Only if the fixed axis is also one of the primary axes does the line of sight describe a plane while moving from one secondary position to another; namely it describes a primary meridian plane.

(5) Transfer of the line of sight directly from one secondary position to another, that is, describing a plane, generally occurs about momentary axes which lie on a conic surface. Only if both secondary positions lie in a primary meridian plane does the rotation occur about a fixed (primary) axis.

Listing gave the rule of orientation without simultaneously providing a proof for it. In its simplest and most elegant form, this proof was given by Helmholtz (9) with the help of the afterimage method. Donders (3) had already found and used the determination of the orientation of the eye with the help of afterimages. This is based on Reute's idea that a vertical afterimage remains vertical on a vertical wall with horizontal sideward turning of the line of sight or vertical raising or lowering, if the eye had been positioned horizontally straight ahead during the recording of the afterimage. In contrast, it leaned with oblique positions of the line of sight. He did not propose a law for these leanings. Wundt (29) also used afterimages for the determination of retinal position, though without coming to a general law. The method of investigation with afterimages will be thoroughly discussed in the next paragraphs, along with the method of Meissner, who first investigated eye position with the help of double images. Fick (7) determined retinal position with the help of the blind spot, a method which Meissner (22) also used later, but which remains significantly behind the other methods in precision.

16. *Determination of Retinal Position with Afterimages*

The determination of retinal positions with afterimages is less exact than investigation with the help of objective images, to be described in the next chapters. It is indispensable in many circumstances, however, and is very useful for an overview, especially in the form given by Helmholtz. I borrow from the latter researcher to set up an experiment proving Listing's Law in the following way.

A large vertically erect wooden frame, divided by an inner cross into four smaller quadrangles, carries a horizontal axis in its middle toward the rear. The frame can be rotated about the axis, which rests on a stand fixed to the wall. On the front the left half of the frame is covered with blue paper and the right with orange paper so that the straight line dividing two colors goes exactly through the point of rotation of the frame. At this point a long fine steel needle is stuck in perpendicular to the plane of the paper, and thus lies exactly in the extension of the axis about which the frame can rotate. Fine lines are placed over the paper parallel to the line dividing the colors except for one line at right angles to the others through the rotation point of the frame. The point of rotation of the frame is at the height of my eyes.

I now place this surface opposite the eye to be investigated so that the fine horizontal needle appears to me in total foreshortening, that is, as a point; I know that the line of sight then meets the plane of the paper perpendicularly. I fixate the needle for some time with unchanging fixation while the dividing line of the colors stands vertical, and then turn my fixation along the horizontal line to the right or left. The originally fixated borderline of the colors then appears to me clear and sharp in an afterimage, and I can compare its direction with the vertical lines which are drawn on the paper. If it always remains parallel to these verticals while fixation deviates to the right or left in an exactly horizontal direction, it proves to me that the eye is rotated about a fixed vertical axis and thus experiences no simultaneous rolling about the line of sight. If a tilting of the borderline visible in the afterimage occurs, the direction of tilting gives me the direction of the rolling of the eyes which has occurred. If I then rotate the frame about its horizontal axis, the originally vertical borderline of the colors with the lines parallel to it appears tilted, and if I again elicit the afterimage it comes to lie on other retinal meridians than before. I now let the eye move along the originally horizontal and now tilted dividing line to one side or the other. I determine by the position of the colored borderline in the afterimage whether the movement of my eye has occurred about a fixed axis perpendicular to its direction and to the line of sight, that is, without rolling, or about momentary axes with simultaneous rolling about the line of sight. In this way, with different positions of the frame I can describe the line of sight to any given direction and convince myself whether a rolling of the eyes has occurred or not.

In order to keep the lines of sight parallel in spite of the relative nearness of the surface, I place a second frame in front of the first and parallel to it. Vertical threads are strung over it so that each has the same distance from its two neighbors as the distance between the middle points of the two eyes. If I erect these parallel lines of sight on the back wall of the surface, I then see the threads singly in spite of the fact that every single one gives me double images. The entire thread system is imaged on identical retinal positions in the right and left eyes even though each pair of identically positioned thread images comes not from one and the same but from two different threads. As soon as the images of the single threads disintegrate into two, it is a sign that the lines of sight are no longer parallel. In this way I can control the parallelism of the lines of sight for every position and movement. However, if the left eye for instance is placed on the point of rotation of the frame and the borderline of the colors is imaged on the vertical retinal meridian, I also receive an image of the color border in the right eye. This, however, is disturbing only when the position of the afterimage approaches the horizontal.

A stable fixing of the head is absolutely necessary to make the experiment exact; the best effort to hold the head still is not adequate because the latter involuntarily follows the eyes in their movements. Because of this, the sensible fixation aligner given by Helmholtz (which will be discussed below) offers no adequate guarantee, although it is a convenient method to assure that the line of sight always has the same position relative to the head when fixation returns to the rotating point of the surface. The head holder which I use is constructed in the following way (figure 16). A horizontal staff about half again as long as the width of the head is fit into two vertical bars so that it can rotate about itself. At its middle, on the upper side, it carries a small board which can be rotated about its vertical axis. This little board has a concave cut on one side, which is coated with a thick layer of shellac as Helmholtz described for his fixation apparatus. The lacquer is softened with warm water and then the little board is grasped with the teeth so that both rows of teeth from above and below make an impression in the lacquer. Every time one again bites the board with the teeth, the latter come exactly into the old impressions and the small board will always have exactly the same position with respect to the head. Or if the board is fixed, the head will have the same position with respect to the board. The two vertical bars are mounted on a heavy stand and can be moved upward

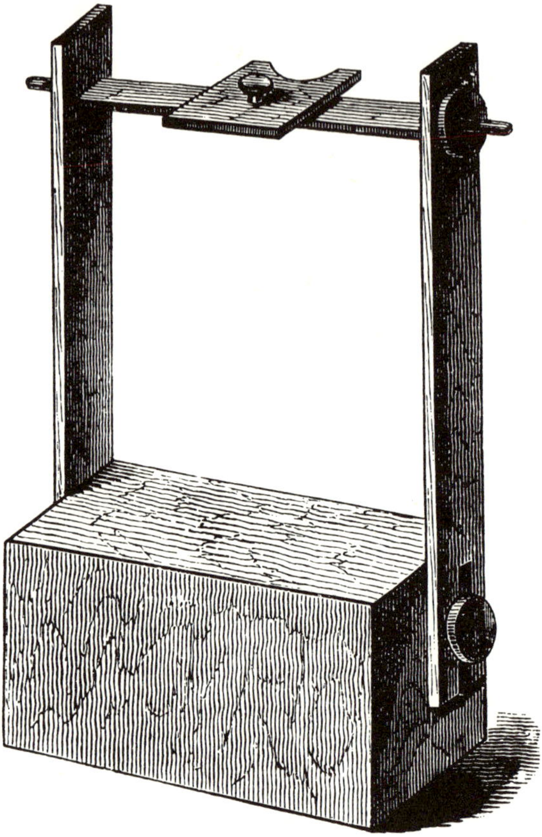

Fig. 16.

and downward. This apparatus is then placed opposite the vertical surface so that the horizontal axis of the apparatus is parallel to the plane of the surface, and when one is fixed on the small board with the teeth, the rotation points of the eyes are at about the same level as the middle of the frame. Now because the small board is rotatable about a vertical axis and the horizontal bar on which it is mounted is rotatable about its own axis, and the latter can be moved up and down by means of the bars which hold it, and finally the entire stand (which is on a small table) is moveable, one can first arrange the apparatus so that the line of sight is exactly perpendicular to the surface if one fixates the point of rotation. And second, without changing this line of sight, one can give the head various positions whereby the eye position relative to the head is changed. If one has found the desired position with the method which I shall describe immediately, then everything can be fixed with screws so that nothing can be misrotated. Whenever one returns to the apparatus and introduces the teeth in the old imprints in the shellac again, one has complete confidence that the head is in exactly the same position relative to the table as before.

Now by trial and error one can find a position of the eyes in which fixation can be moved from the middle point of the vertical surface in a straight line in any direction without the afterimage of the color borderline slanting relative to the parallel lines, provided that these and with them the dividing line of the colors are perpendicular to the direction of eye movement. The eye position determined in this way is therefore the desired primary position. An *exact* agreement of the experimental results with the requirements of Listing's Law will probably never result if the observer has the necessary practice in eliciting sharp afterimages. The move avidly one experiments, however, the more beautiful is the agreement with the Law. One is always more prone to hold two nearly parallel lines for parallel than for not parallel, just as one holds a nearly right angle for a right angle rather than for an oblique one or takes a not quite regular circle for a circle rather than for another curve. These tendencies reduce the effects of not uncommon optical confusions.

In order to find the primary position as quickly as possible, first place the line of sight so that it meets the middle of the surface perpendicularly while the dividing line of the colors stands vertical. One then moves the eyes right and left along the horizontal line on the surface: if the afterimage with the true color borderline begins to diverge upward with these movements, then the eye is too low with respect to the head; if they begin to converge it is too strongly raised. One tilts the head more forward in the first case and more to the back in the latter case, whereby the small tooth board rotates about the horizontal axis. Soon one will find the position for which the afterimage remains parallel with the vertical through all turnings of fixation to the right or left. Now rotate the surface about 90° so that the color borderline comes to lie horizontally and let fixation move up and down along the now-vertical intersecting line. If the afterimage of the borderline now begins to converge to the right with the true borderline, then the line of sight is too far to the right relative to the head; if it begins to converge to the left, then the head is too far to the left. In the first case, one must rotate the head somewhat to the right, in the latter somewhat to the left, whereby the tooth board rotates about the vertical axis. If the board does not happen to have an exactly horizontal position, this rotation axis will not be exactly vertical and one must then again rotate the surface about 90° so that one can again work with the vertical afterimage. Or, one can also begin equally well by eliciting a horizontal afterimage while the board lies exactly horizontal and then go over to the investigation of the vertical afterimage. Every time one somehow misaligns the head one must again observe whether the needle at the point of rotation of the surface still appears in total foreshortening to the fixated eye. In this way one will soon find the position where the vertical afterimage gives the best vertical with horizontal fixation movements, and the horizontal afterimage also remains horizontal to the most exact degree possible with vertical fixation movements. If Listing's Law now applies for the investigated eye, one should be able to give the surface any other desired position without the then-tilted afterimage changing its apparent direction on the surface as one moves fixation in the direction perpendicular to the color borderline.

As long as the line of sight moves in smaller fixation space, Listing's Law has been found until now to be well confirmed for the observer. With peripheral positions of the line of sight all observers find deviations, especially if the line of sight is directed diagonally upward or downward. In addition, one and the same eye never has quite the same primary position; it lies sometimes somewhat higher and sometimes somewhat lower. This is partly because of the inexactness of the method and partly, as Helmholtz has already noted, because the same eye never behaves in exactly the same way.

One's goal is not simply to find the eye position which best expresses the primary position demanded by Listing's Law; on the contrary, one wants to be convinced that the eye does not move strictly according to this Law. To discover the nature of the deviations which occur more or less for every eye, one uses another headholder with the advantage of control of eye position, on which one can read off the present position of the line of sight (figure 17).

Two vertical metal columns are inserted in a mount or on a horizontal table at a distance from one another which is half again as large as the head is wide. Near its upper end each column has a horizontal hole in which a short axle can be rotated; this axle extends beyond the columns on both sides. The axis of one hole lies exactly in the imaginary extension of the other. The inward extending piece of each horizontal axle is vertically drilled through, and through the hole is inserted a vertical brass bar of about 12 centimeters length

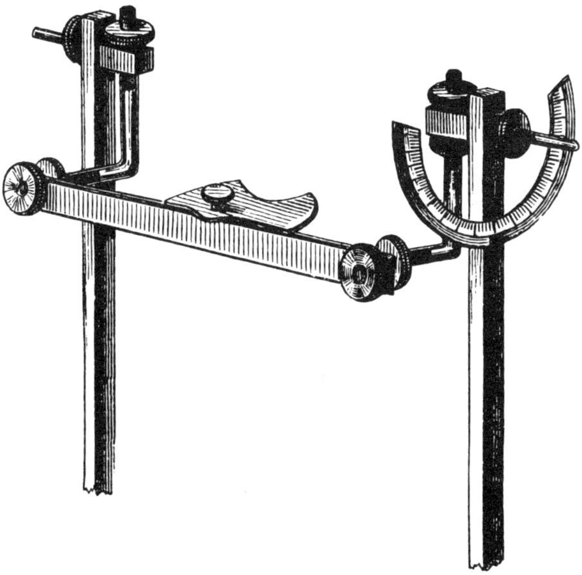

Fig. 17.

whose upper end extends somewhat above the axis. The upper part of this staff is threaded and can be firmly screwed in any desired position by two nuts, one under and the other above the drilled axis. On the lower end of these two vertical brass bars is mounted a thick bar about 8 centimeters in length, directed forward, which therefore forms a perpendicular knee with the vertical bars. The free ends of the horizontal knee joints are also threaded and a horizontal connecting bar with holes is placed on them; the horizontal bar can also be moved forward and backward with two nuts on the horizontal extensions. The horizontal linking bar finally carries a small board with a notch for the teeth. It can be rotated about a vertical axis on the linking bar, can be fixed with a screw, and is otherwise arranged like the headholder described above. If one grasps this small schellac-covered board with the teeth, one can then move the board along with the head fixed to it by screwing the two vertical brass bars up or down; by pushing the linking bar which carries the small board, forward or back, one can move it and with it the head forward or back. And finally, by rotation of the board about its vertical axis, the head can be rotated to the left or right. In this way one can give the head the position in which the line linking the two points of rotation of the eyes falls in exactly the mathematical axis about which the two metal axes rotate in their two columns. Now because these metal axes are bound to the tooth board, which holds the head immobile, one can with the help of this apparatus rotate the head about a line, and with a pointer mounted on the metal axis one can read the nodding of the head (and with it the plane of fixation) on a scale. For instance, if one now holds the head upright, places the fixation plane horizontal, and then nods the head 10° forward, one has moved the fixation plane through 10° while the points of rotation of the two eyes have not been changed.

To control that the points of rotation of the eyes lie in the rotation axis of the apparatus, one brings a vertical surface in front of the head fixed on the small board. Opposite each eye a piece of mirror glass is glued onto the surface with soft wax and a small wooden stick about one inch long is fastened on each of the small mirrors perpendicular to the mirror plane. Through its free end a needle is stuck at right angles. The needle point must lie directly opposite the eye placed horizontally straight ahead. By regulating the somewhat adjustable mirror and the needle in the wax, one can make the fixated needle exactly cover its mirror image. Of course one must choose a distance for the mirror and a separation of the needle from the mirror such that both the needle and its mirror image can be seen fairly sharply at the same time. If one turns his head in the apparatus about the horizontal axis, and thereby just slightly misaligns the point of rotation of the eye (and with it the line of sight of the fixating eye), the needle will no longer cover its mirror image. But with practice one easily finds the position of the tooth board for which the deviation of the mirror image can be brought to a minimum for both eyes. The point which for our purposes can then be taken as the fixed point of rotation of the eyes lies in the axis of the apparatus.

The apparatus appears complicated but when it is once calibrated saves much time and effort, for one can use it for the most varied experiments in which it is useful to exactly control eye position and to know the absolute position of the point of rotation. One can bring before the apparatus a vertical plane parallel to the rotation axis of the apparatus, and mark the two points at which the lines of sight meet the surface perpendicularly when they are horizontal and parallel straight ahead. From a standard position one can then easily calculate the angle of the sideward deviation of the corresponding line of sight for any fixation point to the left or right of these points, since this distance divided by the distance from observation plane to the rotation point of the eyes gives the tangent of the desired angle. Because one can also read the present tilting of the fixation plane from the apparatus, one always knows the exact position of the line of sight relative to the head.

I investigated Listing's Law with my eyes, using the method given by Helmholtz and to be described below in which the head is not fixed. I found that Law to apply for smaller fixation space. But after I had provided a better fixation of the head in the manner described above I succeeded in finding many deviations from this Law, as I had already found with the help of another method (below). Neither of my two eyes moved exactly according to Listing's Law. For both of my eyes, the vertical plane in which I can move the lines of sight by rotating the eyes about a nearly fixed axis perpendicular to the line of sight lies almost exactly parallel to the median plane. The plane in which the eye can move to the left by rotation about a fixed axis within the fixation plane, however, lies higher in both eyes than that in which the line of sight is rotatable to the right about a fixed axis. Specifically, the former plane in my left eye lies about 4° higher than in my right, and the latter in my left eye about 2° higher than my right. In addition, in the left eye the first plane lies about 10° higher than the other and in the right eye only about 8° higher than the other. Between these two planes there is a middle position in both eyes, which (with not quite exact investigation) touches the true primary position of the fixation plane corresponding to Listing's Law. In the left eye this pseudo-primary position of the fixation plane lies slightly higher than in the right. Finally, with all stronger rotations of the eyes, especially in diagonal directions, deviations of no special interest occur.

The numbers given here are averages from many experiments. One definitely does not always obtain the same results, for there are differences of up to 4° in the primary position.

Helmholtz used the visual frame shown in figure 18 for his experiments. A small board with an indentation for the teeth would be grasped by the latter after the edge of the indentation is coated with a layer of soft shellac. On the other end the board carries a small column and on this is glued a bar or a stiff strip of paper pointed on both sides. This strip is exactly as long as the distance between the center points of the two eyes. This can be determined by looking into the distance while one has the small board in the mouth; when the strip is placed parallel to the line of the middle points of the eyes it appears as crossed double images with the two points pointing toward one another, if the strip has the correct length. They will

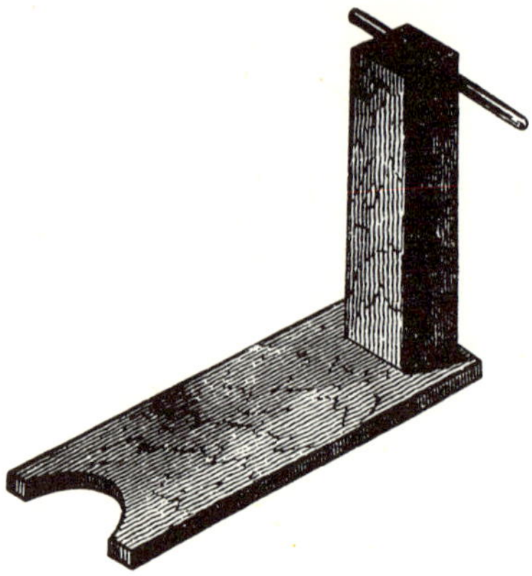

Fig. 18.

overlap one another if the strip is too long or not reach one another if it is too short. Equipped with this visual pointer Helmholtz went before a wall parallel to the facial plane, on which a horizontal colored band was mounted at the height of the eyes for eliciting an afterimage. The lines of sight were now placed horizontally straight ahead with an erect head and at as great a distance as possible, i.e., the band was fixated and the paper strip of the visual pointer was then so arranged that one point of it was in each line of sight. Then the afterimage of the band was elicited and fixation was moved along the band in a horizontal direction. If the afterimage did not remain horizontal and did not continuously cover the true band, the paper strip was moved higher or lower until the primary position of the fixation plane was found. Then fixation would be moved vertically upward or downward; if the afterimage did not remain horizontal, as could be determined by the horizontal lines of the pattern on the wall, the strip would be moved to the right or left far enough that the afterimage remained horizontal with the vertical movement. Whenever the lines of sight were brought back to the middle of the wall in order to freshen the afterimage it could be determined with the help of the pointer that the eyes always had the same position relative to the head; the two points of the paper strip had to cover the fixated point again.

This experiment assumes that when the two eyes are in primary position the lines of sight do not converge noticeably. In any case, the experiment can serve only for a preliminary overview. For more exact investigations Helmholtz used a vertical surface rotatable about its middle point and at the far point of his somewhat shortsighted eyes; on it were a colored paper strip and lines parallel to it. In order to determine that the line of sight of the eye to be investigated was directed at the rotation point of the surface and perpendicular to it, a small mirror in which the eye could see its own pupil was brought to the center of the surface. Here too the visual pointer served to control the head position. Helmholtz found complete agreement with Listing's Law not only with the first method but also with the second, where the observation surface was near the eye. (Helmholtz (15) has recently repeated these experiments with a fixated head and has corroborated Listing's Law in this way as well.)

One can see that the visual pointer controls only the proper positioning of the line of sight relative to the head and the surface, and not various noddings of the head. Further, it controls only the primary position and does not protect against involuntary head rotations with stronger turning of fixation, for which it is necessary to fix the head.

The maximum errors of the afterimage method are fairly large, reaching 1° in the smaller and 2-1/2° in the wider fixation space. I put my head in the holder described above and placed a vertical dial one foot in front of me. It was covered half with blue and half with orange paper so that the dividing line of the two colors ran through the fixed center of the disc. Next to the first dial was a second which could be given any distance from the first. This second dial was covered with gray paper on which a long black strip ran through the middle point. After I had steadily fixated the first dial and had the afterimage of the colored borderline in the eye, I fixated the middle of the second disc and gave myself the task of making the black line on the latter and the colored borderline of the afterimage coincide. The position which I gave to the dial could be read on an indicator. The result was that I did not always place the dial in exactly the same way, which can be explained either by the eye having taken a different orientation each time in spite of equal position of the line of sight or by unsure judgement of the coinciding of the afterimage and the black line. The variability of the position grew with the increase of the sideward distance of the second dial, and the range of the position of the dial reached 5° with the strongest sideward turning of fixation, so that errors up to 2-1/2° were encountered if one assumes that the correct positioning of the dial was exactly in the center of the range of positions.

Further control experiments were done in which the position of the line of sight was not changed at all. A fine black line was drawn through the middle point of the dial covered with colored paper, at right angles to the color borderline. The position of the dial is then read with the help of a scale on the back of the dial, and an afterimage is elicited by steady fixation of the middle point of the dial. Hereupon I gave myself the task of turning the dial far enough that the color border of the afterimage and the black line on the dial covered one another. It happened that I usually did not bring the line exactly into the position that the colored borderline previously had.

An error of 1/4° is very easily made even under the best conditions, that is, when the afterimage is very sharply developed and when the associated eye movements are not at all stressful. Errors of 1/2° are frequent when one has the usual less absolutely sharp afterimage in smaller fixation space. Errors up to 1° are infrequent, though with very difficult eye positions the errors as noted can reach 2-1/2°.

I had already done similar experiments earlier to check Helmholtz's method with unrestrained head and visual pointer. At that time I did not find much larger error ranges than now, with one source of error eliminated by better fixation of the head. Helmholtz wanted to assign the results of this experiment to the stressful convergence position which I had used. But this cannot be a source of error because I placed the objects at approximately the far point of my somewhat short-sighted eyes. Helmholtz further misunderstood my statement that the range of the errors was 2°-5° as though I had said that errors from 2°-5° were made, while I specifically gave these

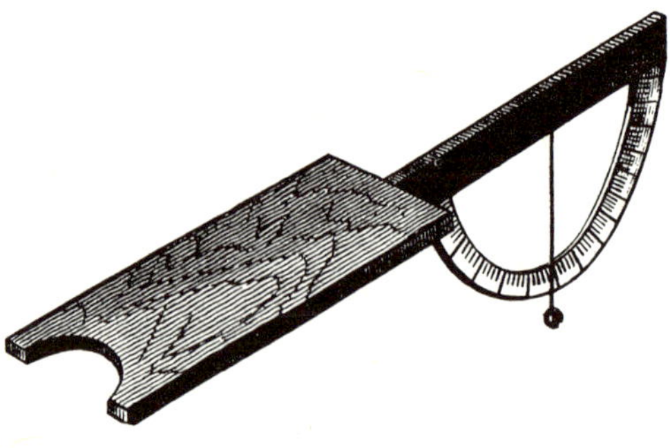

Fig. 19.

numbers only for the range and the errors are only half as large. Helmholtz stated that no errors of over 1/2° occurred. Because he did no control experiments, or at least reported nothing about them, and his method of investigation of eye movements did not permit the elimination of errors through repetition of the experiments, I can take these results to be so much the less generally quanitatively applicable, while I myself have very sharp and lasting afterimages and have many years of experience in experiments with them.

I also add an illustration of a very practical visual pointer given by Berthold (Figure 19), on which one can read either the present nodding of the head from a pendulum, or the angle of the fixation plane if it is always held horizontal with respect to the head.

17. *Determination of Retinal Position with Binocular Images*

The afterimage method has the advantage that it gives us information about any movement of the line of sight and about the position change of each single retina. But because it is indeed not exact enough to answer specific questions which can be asked in the interest of the theory of binocular vision, I have performed my investigations with another method which gives very exact results where the experiments with afterimages are inadequate. I have already described this in its basic outlines (18) and simultaneously indicated small deviations from Listing's Law which I found with it. Later Volkmann and Helmholtz (16) also used this method.

One directs the eyes horizontally straight ahead so that the lines of sight lie parallel, and are perpendicular to a vertical white surface on which two vertical black threads are so suspended that each lies exactly opposite one eye and goes through the point in which the line of sight meets the surface; thus one sees three threads. Specifically, each eye receives two thread-images one of which goes through the point of sight of the retina while the other lies to one side on the retina. The two thread images going through the points of sight fuse for observing into a single thread, which appears in the middle between the other two monocular thread-images. If one now begins to converge slightly, the middle thread image decomposes into two images which indeed do not appear parallel but clearly converge toward the top; this is the only concern of our experiment. But if one rotates the two true threads slightly with the upper end outward and the lower inward, fusion occurs again and splits the single image into two images, again through a slight convergence. These now appear parallel if one has obtained the correct angle of the threads. The two so-called vertical dividing lines (middle longitudinal sections, apparently vertical meridians) diverge by the same angle about which the two true threads diverge at the top, when both retinas diverge upward. If one may further assert that the two vertical dividing lines are now symmetrical to the median plane, half of the observed convergence angle gives us the angular deviation of each of the two dividing lines from the vertical position. But if we know the position of these two retinal meridians, the positions of the two retinas for chosen positions of the lines of sight are also determined.

The afterimage method is of course unable to reveal the position of the vertical dividing lines, but can only give us information about *changes* in their position with any movements of the line of sight. For the theory of binocular vision, however, knowledge of the position of the dividing lines is of greatest importance.

If I do not hold the head upright in the described experiment but nod it forward while the lines of sight remain horizontal and perpendicular to the surface, the divergence of the vertical dividing line grows, that is, I must give the two threads a stronger divergence if the middle thread image is to be broken into two *parallel* images through slight convergence. Conversely, the divergence of the vertical dividing lines decreases if I tilt the head back. If the head is nodded forward in these experiments the fixation plane is raised relative to the head; if the latter is tilted back then the plane is relatively sunken even if its absolute position always remains horizontal. The experiments thus prove that the divergence of the vertical dividing lines grows with raising of the lines of sight in a vertical direction from the so-called primary position, and it shrinks with sinking of the fixation plane. Therefore each eye both with raising and with lowering experiences a rolling about the line of sight which moves the upper end of the vertical dividing line away from the median plane with raising, and brings it closer with sinking. *Listing's Law is therefore not exactly fulfilled for me with purely vertical movements from the primary position.*

The method is as useful for determination of retinal positions with any given sideward directed parallel position as it is for the investigation of symmetrical parallel positions. While it gives us information about the individual position of each eye with symmetrical position, with sideward fixation positions it gives us control only over whether and to what degree the divergence of the two vertical dividing lines changes. It therefore determines only the relative position of the two retinas to one another and not the absolute position of the single retina. This is quite adequate for testing Listing's Law after its general correctness is determined.

More exactly described, my method of investigation was the following. On a horizontal level table a stand holds a vertical surface which reaches down to the table and whose front side is covered with gray paper. The two columns of the headholder described above are screwed into the table in front of the vertical observation surface, which as indicated is so arranged that the head (fixed by the teeth in the apparatus) is rotatable about the horizontal axis through the rotation points of the two eyes. The surface is exactly parallel to this axis and stands for the time being at the far point of my parallel-placed eyes. On it are two long fifteen millimeter wide brass strips, fastened so that the left one lies exactly opposite the left eye and the right one opposite the right eye. Each of the two is rotatable about that point of the surface which lies exactly opposite the point of rotation of the corresponding eye at the same height. The points of rotation of the two brass strips therefore have the same separation as the eyes, and if the lines of sight are placed parallel straight ahead, each meets the opposite strip perpendicularly on the surface at the rotation point. One strip reaches downward, and the other upward nearly to the edge of the surface and carries there a vernier, which slides on a graduated circular frame so that one can read the deviation of the strip from the vertical position with a resolution of minutes. Each strip does not reach as far on the other side in order not to hinder the larger rotations of the strips against one another through excessive length. On the forward side the two strips are covered with the same gray paper as the surface; their two points of rotation are clearly marked with ink. One strip is exactly halved with a white horsehair while the other carries two parallel black horsehairs, one 1 mm to the left and the other 1 mm to the right of the rotation point of the strip. When the two rotation points of the strips fuse binocularly the white hair of one strip appears between the two black ones. The three appear parallel only if the images of the black horsehairs and of the white horsehair fall on parallel retinal meridians on the two retinas. This method of determining retinal position is by far the sharpest of those which I know.

The two points of the table which are perpendicularly under the rotation points of the eyes (l and r in Figure 20) are marked, and from each a straight line (ll' and rr') is drawn to the vertical surface and meets it at a right angle at the lower borderline. In addition to these two lines, which so to say represent the vertical projection of the lines of sight parallel and straight ahead, still other lines radiate out from the points l and r, each deviating 5° from the last. Those going out from one point are made red and the others black. These lines represent the vertical projection of the horizontal fixation plane about the corresponding angle to the left or right. In addition, many lines are drawn sideways, one centimeter apart, parallel to the surface and to the connecting line of the points of rotation on the table. When I want to bring the surface closer or further I can be sure that it always remains parallel to the connecting line of the points of rotation of the eyes. Two small pointers on the lower border of the surface let me simultaneously determine whether the center of the surface has the correct position. The pointers must then meet the table at the lines ll' and rr'. If I then push the surface sideways along a parallel line, when the two pointers meet the two lines on the table which each deviate for instance 10° to the right from the mid-lines ll' and rr' and I again place the lines of sight on the rotation points of the two brass strips, then I know that each line of sight deviates 10° to the right of the median plane. Thus by pushing the surface I can give the lines of sight, which always remain parallel, any desired sideward turning to the left or right, and simultaneously read off the

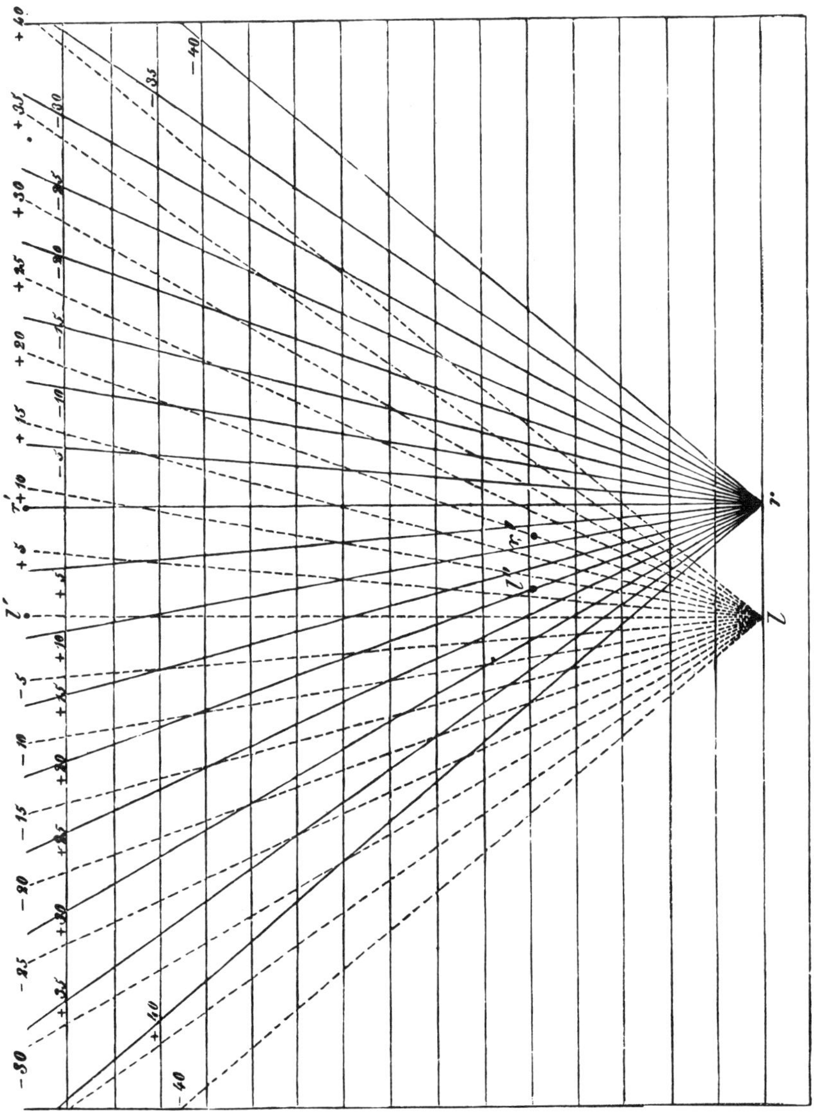

Fig. 20.

degree of sideward turning on the table. If I now tilt the head forward, the pointer on the headholder (see Figure 17) shows me to what degree I have raised or lowered the fixation plane relative to the head. The fixation plane itself always remains horizontal and at right angles to the observation surface, which can move to the right or left with any desired head tilt. Finally, from the position which I must give to the two brass strips so that the three horsehairs appear parallel I can determine the position of the two vertical dividing lines relative to one another. I can then either move both strips out of the vertical position or only one; in the first case I can calculate the divergence angle of the two dividing lines from the sum of the two deviation angles, and in the latter case from the simple deviation angle, that is the angle about which one retina must have been rotated about the line of sight so that both vertical dividing lines lie parallel.

I will call x the angle through which the retina must be cyclorotated in order to bring the thread images in both eyes into corresponding positions. a is the angle through which I must move one brass strip so that the three horsehairs appear parallel, and Φ is the angle of sideward turning of the lines of sight. Thus I find x with the formula $\tan x = \cos \Phi \tan a$. Now if the lines of sight are raised or lowered and turned sideways, the vertical meridians and the primary position are raised or lowered on the median plane according to Listing's Law. The image of the horsehairs now falls on retinal meridians which can deviate several degrees from the vertical dividing line. Thus I do not determine the true divergence of the vertical dividing line by the formula, but the divergence of another pair of identical meridians. For retinas on which the identical meridians are not ordered congruently this can lead to a single merely minimal error. In my eyes this deviation of the positions of the identical meridians from congruence is so small that it does not come into consideration here.

The result of the investigation of parallel positions was that *the divergence angle of the vertical dividing lines of about 2° in the primary position grew with raising of the fixation plane and decreased with its lowering,* as has already been given. *The angle grew, moreover, when the lines of sight were turned to the right or left with unchanged position of the fixation plane, and the growth of the angle with sideward turning was stronger when the fixation plane was more strongly raised.* According to Listing's Law this divergence should always have remained the same. The greatest increase within smaller fixation space, that is, as far as the lines of sight can be held without any strain in the corresponding position, was only 1°; with strenuous holding in sideward rotation it reached 4°. Because the increases were somewhat different for fixations to the left and to the right, as caused by an unequal behavior of my two eyes in their movements, I will not give the resulting numbers. They would have no claim to general validity. Berthold (1) found similar deviations from Listing's Law with sideward turning of the parallel lines of sight and specifically with raised fixation plane in the same sense, but much larger than mine. With lowered fixation plane the deviation was the opposite from mine so that the divergence of the vertical dividing lines decreased. Berthold, however, controlled only the raising or lowering of the fixation plane and not the accompanying position of the head, which as I will show immediately makes small errors possible.

If I turn my parallel lines of sight to the right with strongly raised fixation plane I note that the right line of sight begins to deviate downward, as shown by the appearance of double images lying over one another at the two points which I want to fuse binocularly. The image in the right eye is higher than that in the left. Analogously, the left eye sinks downward if I turn left with raised lines of sight. This holding back downward is stronger when the fixation plane is raised higher and fixation is turned further sidewards. With this position of the lines of sight, the nonparallel direction specifies a change in the divergence of the vertical dividing lines according to Listing's Law, and the observed divergence angle gives us no measure for the deviation from Listing's Law. If one now does not fix the head, one has a small involuntary rotation of the head such that the eye moved downward is slightly raised, and double vision ceases although the lines of sight are still not in a single plane. Thus one receives false divergences if one performs such experiments with only one visual pointer and without a firmly fixed head.

The divergence of the vertical dividing lines with symmetrical parallel position of the lines of sight, which I have noted previously (17), has been found earlier; Helmholtz (8, 10) has found it independently. Helmholtz has also found the above discussed deviation from Listing's Law with vertical raising and sinking of the parallel lines of sight, with the help of the same method. It appears that this deviation is the rule, although its degree is very variable. With my eyes the divergence of the vertical dividing lines grow to nearly 1-1/2° if I transfer from the deepest possible symmetrical parallel position to the highest. For Helmholtz it grew only 1/3° and for Berthold (1) much more.

I will now describe a few preparations which allow an improvisation to prove the result just described. A wood or cardboard screen which is white on one side is mounted vertically parallel to the facial plane. Exactly opposite one eye a small hole is poked perpendicularly through the screen and on the side opposite the face some soft wax is pressed over the opening. Now from behind one sticks a small long and exactly straight needle, for instance an insect needle, through the wax and the hole, applies a square to it from several sides and thus positions it perpendicular to the front screen surface by pushing in the soft wax from behind. If one already knows the distance between the two middle points of his eyes when placed parallel, then a second needle is placed perpendicular to the screen surface at this horizontal distance from the first. If one does not know this distance, or wants to make the apparatus simultaneously usable for other eyes which have a somewhat different distance from one another, he makes an approximate estimate of the distance between the eyes and makes a small horizontal slit for the second needle opposite the second eye; on closing that eye the first needle appears in total foreshortening, that is its center is the center of a small area. Then without moving the head one pushes the second already perpendicular needle trailwise back and forth in the slot until it appears in total foreshortening to the now open eye with closing of the first eye. One then fixes the second needle with wax as well. After alternate testing of the left and right needles one will quickly arrive at this goal with a little skill.

On the front side of the screen one suspends two fine plumb lines discernible by the colors of their threads so that each touches one needle at its insertion point. One can fix the threads above and weight them with a small weight below. One now places his head so that each eye sees the needle on its side in total foreshortening, that is, with closing of the other eye. One then fixates the middle between the two needles without moving the head in the slightest, then reduces the convergence of the eyes and pays attention to the double images of the two threads which are approaching one another while ignoring the other two double images which are diverging from one another. If the lines of sight are nearly parallel, one clearly notes the convergence of the thread images upward.

Each eye naturally receives two images with such eye positions, one of which is seen directly while the other appears indirectly sideward and is not considered here.

The screen must of course be brought to a distance at which the threads and needles can be seen clearly enough in spite of the parallel positioning of the eyes. Slight shortsightedness is best suited to this; normal sighted people must use either a larger and more distant screen or lenses, whose somewhat disturbing influence should be noted.

I assert that the experimenter can voluntarily move his eyes to a parallel position in spite of the nearness of the screen. This will present no difficulty for those with practice in stereoscopy with free eyes, and if necessary one can place a tube in front of each eye.

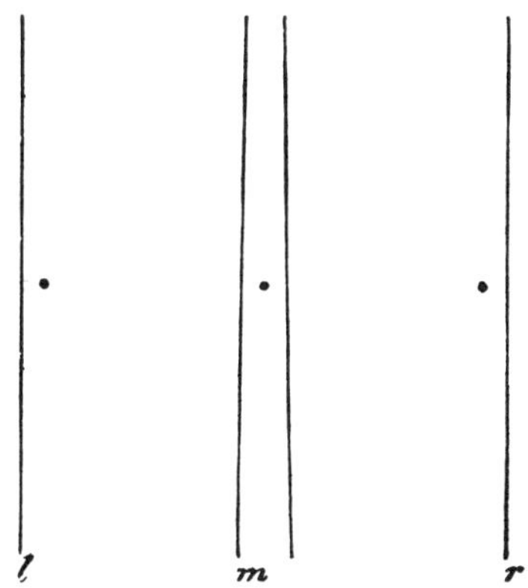

Fig. 21.

One now lets the two threads go not through the lines of sight but somewhat outward from them, while the points at which the lines of sight meet the surface are sharply marked, and places the lines of sight not on the threads but on the points. One then sees a single point between two very close threads (*m* in Figure 21) where the latter do indeed converge upward and are parallel only if the threads have retinal images parallel to the vertical dividing lines with an appropriate divergence. The observation with exactly parallel lines of sight can also be arranged here, and it is not necessary to first divide the fused image of the threads with a slight convergence, which always brings a slight inexactness with it. But it is difficult for the unpracticed to focus the lines of sight on the points; they are much more likely to place them on the lines and then see only one line but two points. This unfortunate situation can be minimized if one makes the threads of different colors.

Helmholtz did not use two threads of the same color on a contrasting background, but colored the surface white on one half and black on the other and stretched a black thread over the first half and a white one over the second. For those for whom the voluntary parallel positioning of the lines of sight is easy, this is strongly recommended; for others it makes the parallel positioning more difficult because of the dissimilarity of the two threads to be fused. Helmholtz further used a straight-bordered red strip of three millimeters width instead of a thread and gave a blue thread to the other eye, both on black backgrounds. The thread had to appear in the middle line of the red stripe. This is also recommended for those who have good control over their eyes.

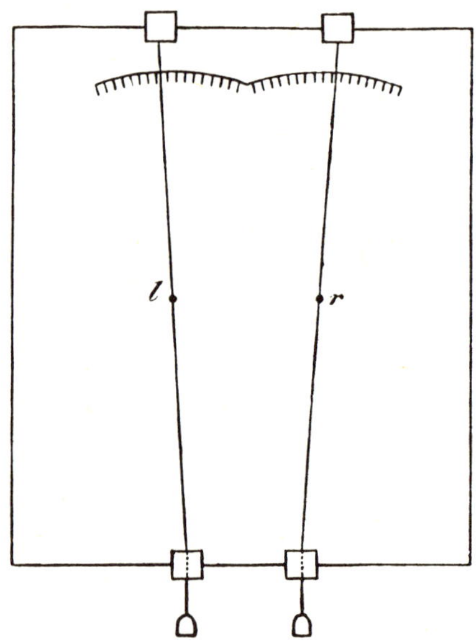

Fig. 22.

In order to easily regulate and determine the divergence of the threads, one can set a moveable rider on the upper edge of the surface (Figure 22) on which the thread is fastened. On the under edge of the surface one similarly places a small indicator which is vertically drilled through so that the thread, weighted at the bottom, can be led through it. Two arcs are drawn through the points of sight *l* and *r* of the two eyes and are graduated so that one can read the deviations of the two threads from the vertical position. Of course the threads must always be spanned in a straight line over the surface and may not be bent about the two vision needles at *l* and *r* but must just graze them. Still another method deserves description; in its important aspect it has already been used by von Recklinghausen (25), as I have described earlier (17), and has also recently been used by Volkmann, as Helmholtz has communicated on the basis of a letter. With this method the observation lines do not go through the two points of sight but begin at them and run radially, one upward and the other downward. For instance, at the two points at which the lines of sight meet the described vertical surface, one thread (contrasting well with the color of the table) is fastened at one end for each point. The free end of one thread is inserted through the vertical hole of an indicator on the bottom edge of the surface and weighted with a small weight, while the free end of the other thread goes through the vertical hole in an indicator on the upper edge of the surface and hangs weighted by a weight behind the surface as shown in Figure 23. If one wants to omit the slide indicators one can also fix the threads in the proper positions with nails. The two arcs in the arrangement shown in the figure permit reading of the angle about which each thread deviates from the vertical direction.

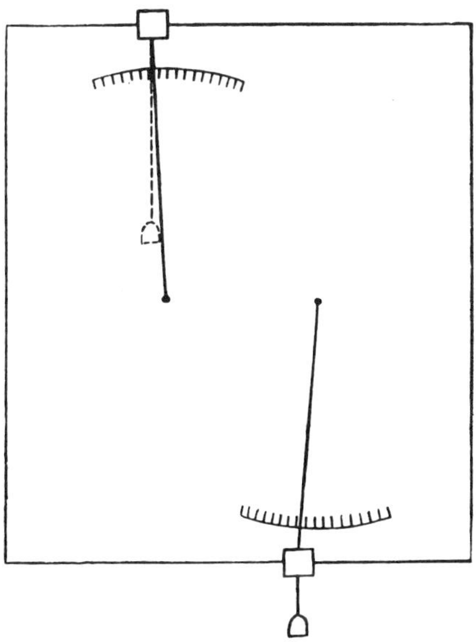

Fig. 23.

If one orients the lines of sight in the described way after one has marked the points *l* and *r* well, then the latter fuse to an apparently single point. The two threads fuse together to an apparently single thread going over the entire surface, and their middle point appears bent if the two threads lie in the true vertical. But if one pushes the two slides somewhat to the left, then the threads appear straight when the deviation of the true threads from the vertical is exactly as large as the deviation of their vertical dividing line. Of course, one can also orient the threads in a horizontal direction or any other direction instead of the vertical. Berthold worked with this method with horizontal threads. Like Volkmann one can also use lines which are radially arranged on small dials instead of threads. But because the radius of these dials may be only as large as half the interocular distance, this modification is appropriate only for the shortsighted if one does not want to use convex glasses. Radial divisions also cannot be made on the dial because the divisions would otherwise be too fine. Rather, one must make other further arrangements to be able to read the current rotation on an arc scale of a larger radius.

18. *Investigation of Retinal Position with Converging Lines of Sight*

Meissner (23) was the first to investigate the cyclorotary position of the retinas with different and especially with symmetrical convergence positions. He began with the observation that if one fixates a point behind or in front of the plane, a line in the median plane and vertical to the fixation surface appears in parallel double images only at a quite specific tilt of the fixation plane to the head. If the fixation plane is relatively higher, the double images diverge upward, and if they are crossed, the fixation plane lies relatively lower and the crossed double images converge upward. One can make the double images parallel by tilting the observation line with its upper end away from the head in the first case or toward the head in the latter case. From the acute angle which the observation line makes with the fixation plane, and from the convergence angle of the lines of sight, Meissner then sought to calculate the angle between the vertical dividing line and the fixation plane. This method is useful in principle, but the way in which Meissner used it contains several sources of error which I have specified earlier (17). Because Meissner did not yet know that even with parallel lines of sight the vertical dividing lines do not lie parallel, he drew the conclusions from his observations that the lines of sight find themselves in Listing's primary position if they deviate 45° downward from their horizontal position.

I have performed the experiment of convergence positioning analogously to the parallel positioning, and therefore have not elicited double images of a single line, but again used a single line in one eye and two parallel lines in the other. I then arranged the lines of sight and regulated the relative tilts of the observation lines so that one line appeared to me exactly in the middle between the two others, and these appeared parallel. At the same time I have always experimented with a horizontal visual plane and a vertical observation plane. In this way all sources of error in Meissner's method are eliminated.

The apparatus described in the above paragraphs needs only a small change for this. The two brass strips which carried the observation lines were brought close enough together that they stood only half the distance of the rotation points of the two eyes from one another. If I now place the left line of sight on the rotation point of the right and the right on that of the left brass strip, then I can again proceed quite analogously as with the parallel position. Perpendicularly under the rotation points of each stripe the surface had one mark for each on its lower edge; these marks, which gave the sideward deviations of the lines of sight in degrees, were arranged in the described way on the radiating lines of the table. Thus, if for instance the left mark came to lie exactly on the radius marked +20° on the right radiating system, and the right mark on the +20° mark of the left radiating system (Figure 20, *l''*, *r''*), then I was sure that both of my lines of sight converged by about 40° as long as I focused the left line of sight on the rotation point of the right and the right on the rotation point of the left brass strip in this way. The observation surface can always remain parallel to the frontal surface, and the conversion of the angles is simplified. Thus the lines of sight cross in front of the surface with this observation method, and the observed objects lay behind their crossing point. At the same time the distance of the surface from the crossing point of the lines of sight was small enough to permit a sharp perception of the lines, especially because long practice had weakened the usually strict dependence between accommodation and convergence in my eyes. Otherwise I would have been free to move the two brass strips even closer to one another, or with weaker convergence angles to focus the left line of sight on the left strip and the right on the right, so that the intersection point of the lines of sight would have been behind the surface.

With the strongest convergence angles the two brass strips would again have the original distance of the rotation points of the eyes. The crossing point of the lines of sight is therefore only half as far from the eyes as it is from the surface. Sharp vision was still possible for me in spite of this only because with these stronger convergences accommodation generally begins to lag behind convergence. Aside from this, the larger distance of the strips from one another made it possible to create very strong convergences of the lines of sight here without bringing the surface too near to the headholder. In general, the method permits changing of the distance between the strips according to one's requirements without making necessary a conversion of the observation data, for one can read the deviations of each line of sight on the radiating lines of the surface.

For simplicity I have always left the brass strip fixated by the left eye in the vertical position during my experiments, and I have given the other strip the deviation necessary for an apparent parallelism of the observation threads. In this way I could determine the angle which the fixation plane in the right eye made with that retinal meridian in the left eye which appeared identical to the plane lying vertical to the fixation plane. This angle indicated about how many degrees the right eye would have to be cyclorotated to create a corresponding position of both retinas.

In table 2 below I have displayed the results of several series of experiments. One sees three columns divided with heavy lines, of which each again consists of three sub-columns. Each first sub-column contains the angle by which the vertical dividing lines deviate from the position vertical to the fixation plane with ten, twenty, or thirty degrees of inward turning of both eyes, that is twenty, forty, or sixty degrees of convergence. If they deviate with the upper end outward the angles are indicated as positive and in the opposite case as negative. The angles given are therefore the so-called circular rotation (Raddrehung) angles of Helmholtz. These are calculated according to the formula $\tan x = \tan a \cos\Phi$ from the angles read from the table, where a is read from the table, Φ is the deviation angle of the line of sight inward, and x is the desired angle. Each second sub-column gives the angle about which the vertical dividing line must deviate from the perpendicular to the fixation plane if the eye has that orientation which Listing's Law specifies for the corresponding position of the lines of sight. Here the primary position of my fixation plane is taken as that position which best corresponds to the demands of Listing's Law as it has been discussed above. In addition the angle through which each vertical dividing line deviates from vertical in the primary position is set at one degree.

Each third sub-column, finally, gives the angle about which the observed position of the dividing line deviates from the calculation according to Listing's Law. This angle is indicated as positive when the vertical dividing line deviated with its upper end outward, as was almost always the case, and as negative if it deviated inward from the position predicted by Listing's Law.

The table shows *that in general the vertical dividing lines with symmetrical convergence are tilted with their upper ends further outward and correspondingly less inward than Listing's Law would predict, and that this (positive) deviation grows very quickly on the one hand with increase of the convergence angle and on the other hand with lowering of the fixation plane.* Only with a raised visual plane and with small convergence angles (20°) do we find a small deviation in the opposite (negative) sense, that is, the vertical dividing lines are tilted outward less than one would expect according to Listing's Law. The lowest row of figures shows how significant the deviations from Listing's Law can be. With lowering of the fixation plane of 50°, the deviation from Listing's Law at a convergence angle of 20° is almost 3° for each eye; with a convergence angle of 40° it is almost 4° and with a convergence of 60° almost 6°.

The results of these experiments were that the law which applies for far positions does not apply for near positions, and that with stronger convergences of the lines of sight the deviations from that law are so large that it loses all applicability for near vision. I have done many series of experiments but do not find it useful to

Table 2

Convergence Angle	20°			40°			60°		
Angle of inward turning of each line of sight	10°			20°			30°		
Tilt of the fixation plane	observed	calculated	difference	observed	calculated	difference	observed	calculated	difference
+15°	+2° 1′	+2° 19′	–0° 18′						
+10°	+1° 46′	+1° 53′	–0° 7′	+3° 34′	+2° 46′	+0° 48′			
+ 5°	+1° 30′	+1° 26′	+0° 4′	+3° 22′	+1° 53′	+1° 29′	+6° 17′	+2° 21′	+3° 56′
0°	+1° 21′	+1°	+0° 25′	+3° 25′	+1°	+2° 15′	+4° 47′	+1°	+3° 47′
– 5°	+1° 14′	0° 34′	+0° 40′	+2° 46′	+0° 7′	+2° 39′	+4° 3′	–0° 21′	+4° 24′
–10°	+1° 7′	+0° 7′	+1°	+1° 50′	–0° 46′	+2° 36′	+3° 2′	–1° 41′	+4° 43′
–15°	+0° 59′	–0° 19′	+1° 18′	+1° 11′	–1° 40′	+2° 51′	+1° 53′	–3° 2′	+4° 55′
–20°	+0° 52′	–0° 46′	+0° 38′	+0° 35′	–2° 34′	+3° 9′	+0° 52′	–4° 25′	+5° 17′
–25°	+0° 42′	–1° 13′	+1° 55′	+0° 10′	–3° 29′	+3° 39′	–0° 9′	–5° 48′	+5° 39′
–30°	+0° 28′	–1° 41′	+2° 9′	–0° 38′	–4° 25′	+3° 47′	–1° 29′	–7° 13′	+5° 44′
–35°	+0° 10′	–2° 10′	+2° 20′	–1° 25′	–5° 22′	+3° 57′	–2° 49′	–8° 39′	+5° 50′
–40°	0°	–2° 39′	+2° 39′	–2° 2′	–6° 21′	+4° 19′	–4° 16′	–10° 8′	+5° 52′
–45°	–0° 23′	–3° 8′	+2° 45′	–3° 15′	–7° 22′	–4° 7′			
–50°	–0° 43′	–3° 40′	+2° 57′	–1° 30′	–8° 24′	–3° 54′			

give averages because these would have meaning only if I could generalize from at least twenty experimental series. The single results are specifically dependent upon chance occurrences, as I have already indicated above with far positions. Orientation varies slightly with one and the same fixation position, if one fixates the same point for a long time or in general tires specific muslces. The order in which one performs the experiments is also important. In this one can proceed as one will; each experimental series contains the same laws and these express themselves so clearly and concern such large angles that observational differences of several minutes, and with stronger convergences even of half a degree, cannot obscure the lawfulness of the numbers found in the series. I would have pursued the experiments further if the motor inequality of my two eyes had not occurred even more than with far positions. It would be most interesting if someone whose eyes behave completely symmetrically in a motor sense and who had the necessary practice in such experiments could further follow experimentally the important questions given here. But one should not believe that these small deviations of my eyes from symmetry could influence the results given below enough that one could not take these as an expression of a generally applicable law. Namely, these deal partly with very large numbers and partly with observations of other researchers which adequately prove that this law is generally applicable.

If Listing's Law also applied for near positions, then the lines of sight could converge to any degree in the primary visual plane, and the retinal meridians which are vertical in the primary position would remain vertical in all convergence positions; each vertical dividing line would therefore deviate about 1° from the vertical position as before. With a raised fixation plane, according to Listing's Law, every originally vertical meridian would tip with its upper end outward as soon as the lines of sight symmetrically converged, and would do so more strongly the higher the convergence angle on the one hand and the greater the raising of the fixation plane on the other. The vertical dividing lines, because they are already tilted with their upper ends outward with parallel lines of sight, would tilt correspondingly more strongly outward in the eye positions described as the lines of sight converged. This tilting would grow both with convergence of the lines of sight and with raising of the fixation plane. On the other hand, with lowered fixation plane the vertical dividing lines would turn with their upper ends inward, and thus with weak convergence would approach the position vertical to the fixation plane. With increasing convergence or lowering they would go through this vertical position and would then tilt against the fixation plane with the upper ends inward. If we now compare the experimentally found positions of the vertical dividing lines with those calculated from Listing's Law, we generally find significant deviations in the sense that the dividing lines are tilted more strongly with the upper ends outward and correspondingly less inward than the law would indicate; these deviations from the law increase rapidly as convergence increases.

Thus if I fixate a near point N with a tilting of the fixation plane of 50° under a convergence of 60°, and over the right eye, and then direct my attention to a far point F (which also lies on the unmoved line of sight of the left eye), then the eye rolls about the line of sight as it accommodates for distance such that the upper end of the meridian previously vertical to the fixation plane goes inward. If I accommodate again for the near object N, the eye experiences a rolling about the line of sight in the opposite direction, in both cases of 5°.

This rolling about an unchanged line of sight can also be easily made clear with an afterimage. For instance, bring a vertical colored strip of paper to the location of the far point F in the discussed location of the left line of sight and elicit an afterimage. A vertical pane of glass stands before the eye at the distance of the point N, which is marked on a vertical line at the location of the point. Then accommodate for the latter point. The afterimage will not appear vertical on the pane of glass but will be tilted through the point N with its upper end outward, that is, deviated to the left for the left eye. In general one can investigate the orientation of the retinas at near positions with the afterimage method and must only experiment binocularly with them so that the afterimage is elicited in just one eye, while the fixation point with near vision would be visible with both eyes. I had already begun these experiments once, but had to give them up at that time because my eyes were already very strained by much experimentation. It is especially difficult to keep the afterimage alive with strong convergence of the lines of sight because each large muscular effort of the eyes weakens the afterimage. Very intensive afterimages are therefore necessary for these experiments. At present I am not in a condition to take up these experiments again because my eyes have many demands on them from other investigations. Only this much can be given as an important result: if I deviate one eye significantly from the primary position, and then with unchanged line of sight strongly accommodate for nearness, a striking rotation of the originally vertical afterimage occurs such that its upper end tilts inward, while with turning of the eye inward an opposite rotation of the afterimage occurs in agreement with the facts given above. *Therefore, during accommodation for nearness the inward turned eye with unchanged line of sight experiences a cyclorotation with the upper part outward, and the outward turned eye experiences a rolling inward, while the other line of sight is forced to deviate inward,* as has been discussed earlier.

I have also investigated asymmetrical convergence positions in the manner discussed above. In these experiments when the fixation point was to the left of the median plane I received somewhat larger deviations than when it was to the right, a result of the somewhat unequal motility of my two eyes. In general, these experiments can say nothing about the absolute position of each single retina because of the asymmetrical position of the lines of sight. They can only instruct us about the position of one with respect to the other. The angle about which one retina appears rotated about the line of sight generally does not change very greatly when fixation is turned sideward with constant convergence angle. As the afterimage experiments just described show, this is related to the convergence-dependent deviation from Listing's Law where the effect on an eye turned outward can be opposite to that on one which is turned inward. For reasons already given, I will omit the individual results of these experiments.

These experiments thus show that Donder's Law, according to which the orientation of the eye should depend solely on the position of the line of sight, does not have a general validity, but rather that retinal position is determined by the position of the point of sight, which can vary with unchanged position of one line of sight. They further show that Listing's Law for the positions and movements of the eyes does not apply for near vision, and they finally reveal that innervation for the purpose of near vision is not restricted to the adductors and focus muscles but also extends to other extraocular muscles. With the sparse observations which are available up to now it is still impossible to determine the muscles whose activity is associated with the adductors of the double eye.

It would be of great interest to know these muscles, and further to know whether they are always the same whether the fixation plane is raised or lowered. If any facts at all were available which would indicate that a general tension of the extraocular muscles could facilitate accommodation for nearness, as has frequently been assumed earlier, then one could find a further proof of such a relationship in the observed change of orientation with accommodation for nearness.

It would appear that we have become accustomed to a specific deviation from Listing's Law for every orientation of the eye in the interest of clear vision (see Chapter 19). But I cannot automatically agree with this assumption because the deviation from Listing's Law also occurs with fixation positions which we never use in ordinary vision. One must therefore limit this hypothesis to the extent that we have accustomed ourselves once and for all to use one orientation-correcting innervation whenever we want near vision, no matter what the position of the fixation plane. That the effect of this innervation appears different in various fixation positions could be determined purely mechanically by the changed positions of all the muscles, as indeed the involuntary convergence of the lines of sight with lowering of the fixation plane also has a purely mechanical origin (as was proved above).

The indicated orientation of the double eye at its near position is not idiosyncratic, for the conclusion can be drawn even now from the sparse material which is available in the work of others that we are concerned here with a quite generally applicable behavior. Here the investigation of Meissner already referred to deserves a review. He found that with a lowering of the fixation plane of about 45° from the horizontal position, a fixated line in the median plane perpendicular to the fixation plane was imaged on identical retinal meridians for any desired convergence, i.e., on the vertical dividing lines. From this he concluded that the lines of sight lowered forty-five degrees and parallel to the median plane were in Listing's primary position. In fact, his results entitled him to the conclusion that if he rolled both eyes inward from this assumed primary position simultaneously about equal angles, with unchanged fixation plane, then the rotation of the eyes occurred about a fixed axis at right angles to the fixation plane and to the lines of sight. Now Meissner's method had several sources of error, which as I have pointed out elsewhere are not of a kind that make the results of his experiments useless for our purposes. It can be assumed with much greater certainty that in Meissner's eye the vertical dividing line in the specified position of the fixation plane is indeed very nearly if not exactly vertical to the fixation plane. If we compare this fact with the results of my experiments, it is shown that my eyes behave very similarly with a lowering of the fixation plane of about 25° from the primary position as Meissner's do with a lowering of about 45° from the horizontal position. When my lines of sight converge between 40° and 60° with this fixation position, my vertical dividing lines do indeed lie nearly vertical to the fixation plane, while with a convergence angle of 20° I must lower the fixation plane even further so that the vertical dividing lines come to this position. One would think thereby that the numbers given by me are not averages, but are burdened with all of the chance errors of a simple experimental series, and that we do not know at all whether the position of the fixation plane which Meissner observed as the horizontal corresponds to the primary position of his fixation plane. Because it cannot be immediately assumed that Meissner's eyes did not deviate significantly from the directions of Listing's Law with far vision from his later experiments, it follows that with near vision his eyes show deviations from the law analogous to mine. In the following table, in which I have indicated the calculated deviations of the vertical dividing lines according to Meissner's results, the same law is apparent as in the deviations which I found. (Meissner has calculated his experimental data according to an inexact formula which, however, specifies only small errors and always in the same direction. I have considered it superfluous to recalculate all of Meissner's corresponding numbers but give them in table 3 as he gives them.) I have indicated as positive the angle about which the vertical dividing lines deviated from the position vertical to the fixation plane with the upper end outward.

For our purposes table 3 would naturally have greater value if Meissner's primary position were known. But his primary fixation plane probably would not deviate significantly from the 0° position indicated in the table. We also do not know how much tilting of the vertical dividing lines to the fixation plane Meissner already showed in the primary position. In spite of this, the table shows that the vertical dividing lines deviate at all convergence positions with the upper ends outward from the position which they must have according to Listing's Law. At the 0° position of the fixation plane the lines of sight are deviated about 3° and the vertical dividing lines deviate about 0°45′ outward. This deviation grows to 3° when the inward deviation of the lines of sight increases to 20°. Similarly, we find with raising or lowering of the fixation plane by about 20° that the deviations of the vertical dividing lines still grow if convergence increases. But now the primary position of the fixation plane is contained in the region between 20° raising and 20° lowering, from which it follows that Meissner's eyes, like mine, experience a rolling with the upper part outward when the lines of sight converge symmetrically in the primary fixation plane. The deviation from Listing's Law occurs more and more strongly just as in my eyes, whether one assumes the primary position to be the one indicated as 0° or a deeper one. As long as one has the opinion that the eye moves according to the same laws with distant vision as with near vision, Meissner's results would be nearly inconceivable if one did not assume quite extraordinary individual differences.

We must thank von Recklinghausen for a second larger series of

Table 3

Convergence angle	5° 56′	7° 38′	9° 16′	11° 48′	13° 10′	14° 52′	20° 2′	22° 38′	28° 4′	33° 24′	35° 4′	41° 6′
Angle of inward turning of each line of sight	2° 58′	3° 49′	4° 38′	5° 54′	6° 35′	7° 26′	10° 1′	11° 19′	14° 2′	16° 42′	17° 32′	20° 33′
Tilt of the fixation plane +40°						+3° 12′						+8° 15′
+30°						+2° 46′			+4°			+5° 4′
+20°						+2° 22′			+3° 10′			+4° 11′
+10°						+1° 50′			+2° 20′			+3° 28′
0°	+0° 45′	+0° 16′	+0° 50′	+1° 6′	+1° 25′	+1° 43′	+1° 45′	+1° 47′	+2° 1′	+2° 15′	+2° 26′	+3° 2′
−10°	+0° 28′	+0° 30′	+0° 36′	+0° 49′	+1° 5′	+1° 20′	+1° 7′	+1° 15′	+1° 20′		+1° 37′	+2° 4′
−20°	+0° 10′	+0° 14′	+0° 22′	+0° 36′	+0° 39′	+0° 51′	+0° 36′	+0° 39′	+0° 42′		+1° 50′	+1° 22′
−30°	0°	0°	+0° 9′	+0° 17′	+0° 26′	+0° 35′	+0° 35′	+0° 38′	+0° 38′		+0° 46′	+0° 41′
−40°	0°	0°	0°	+0° 4′	+0° 7′	+0° 18′	0°	0° 4′	0°		0°	0°
−45°	0°	0°	0°	0°	0°	0°	0°	0°	0°		0°	0°
−50°						0°		−0° 20′	−0° 40′			−0° 41′
−60°						−0° 22′		−2°	−1° 30′			

experiments with symmetrical positions. He experimented with a line in the visual plane parallel to the baseline, which was bent around its middle point so that both of its halves could be raised or lowered about the same angle over the fixation plane while the point of the angle so constructed always remained in the fixation plane. In the median plane he arranged a screen which reached to the middle point of the line so that each eye saw only half of the line when its middle point was binocularly fixated. From the angle about which each half-line had to be raised or lowered so that the line was no longer bent but appeared straight he could calculate the angle about which the horizontal dividing line deviated from the fixation plane. In table 4 I have indicated the results of his experiments. Again, the deviation angles are positive when the outer end of the horizontal dividing line is below the fixation plane. It is irrelevant for our purposes that Recklinghausen used the horizontal instead of the vertical dividing line. From the table the same law is again apparent.

Finally, results which Helmholtz has recently reported in his *Physiological Optics* are to be reviewed. He informs us on the basis of letters that Volkmann, with a point 30 centimeters away and lying in the horizontal fixation plane, found an increase of the divergence of the vertical dividing lines of both eyes of 2°. This compares with the difference which the respective meridians should have according to Listing's Law. With increasing convergence this deviation grew for Volkmann as well, and he also observed small rotations of an after-image when he strongly changed accommodation. We must await the individual data of the experiments and their more exact description to be able to judge these reports. Using another method which was practically the same as Recklinghausen's, Helmholtz found that with symmetrical convergence on a point 21 centimeters away and in the primary position of the fixation plane, there is a deviation from Listing's Law of 0° 17′, in the same direction as for the other observers. With afterimages he also observed that when the line of sight deviated strongly sidewards, a deviation of the afterimage of 2° to 2°30′ appeared with convergence and was in the same direction as I have given above. With inward turning of the eye the upper ends of the vertical dividing lines move outward; with turning of the eyes outward they move in the opposite sense, as though, as he says, the primary position for the convergence positions were deeper than for parallel positions. The latter assumption would not apply badly for my eyes. Dastich, as Helmholtz reports, is supposed to have found no influence of convergence at all. The methods of the investigation and the convergence angle used are not given, however. Schuurmann found (as I reported according to Helmholtz because I do not have the original work) that with afterimage experiments no rolling occurs through Donders' conversions, but on the contrary rollings of 1° to 3° occur with extreme convergences.

Table 4

Convergence angle	15° 50′	18° 12′	20° 44′	24° 6′	25° 44′	27° 40′	29° 52′	32° 26′	35° 30′	37° 14′	39° 8′	41° 16′	43° 36′	42° 14′	49° 8′
Inward turning of each line of sight	7° 55′	9° 6′	10° 22′	12° 3′	12° 52′	13° 50′	14° 56′	16° 13′	17° 45′	18° 37′	19° 34′	20° 38′	21° 48′	23° 7′	24° 34′
Tilt of the fixation plane															
+40°		+3° 2′						+4° 41′							
+30°	+0° 56′	+1° 41′	+2° 2′		+2° 33′	+2° 49′		32′	+1°	+4° 10′			+5° 6′		
+20°	+0° 50′	+1° 2′	+1° 23′	+1° 54′		+2° 7′	+2° 19′	+2° 32′	+2° 55′		+3° 16′		+3° 41′	+3° 59′	
+10°	+0° 35′	+0° 56′		+1° 33′		+1° 48′	+1° 52′	+1° 59′	+2° 5′		+2° 4′		+2° 38′	+2° 58′	
0°	+0° 21′		+0° 30′			+0° 39′	+0° 46′	+1° 1′	+1° 20′	+1° 33′		+1° 50′		+2° 10′	
−10°	+0° 18′	+0° 27′	+0° 42′			+0° 51′		+0° 58′			+1° 14′		+1° 31′		+1° 56′
−20°	+0° 15′	+0° 24′		+0° 36′		+0° 39′			+0° 52′			+1° 3′			
−30°	0°	+0° 15′					+0° 34′		+0° 22′				30° 47′		
−35°	0°	0		0		0	0	0	0		0		0		0
−40°	−0° 6′	0	0	0		−0° 18′	−0° 18′	−0° 21′	−0° 37′		−0° 53′				−1° 1′
−50°	−0° 18′		−0° 27′		−0° 50′				−1° 38′		−1° 55′				−2° 57′
−60°	−0° 38′		−0° 48′		−1° 30′				−2° 18′	−2° 41′					
−70°					−3° 21′										

19. *On the Optical Meaning of the Orientation Laws*

It is clear that the motor apparatus of the visual organ must match its sensory apparatus as the shell does the egg. Whether one assumes that both are arranged according to a wise plan, or that they have developed with one another and through one another in naturally necessary ways through the animal series, in any case the capabilities of one must bespeak the demands of the other. It follows that the eye muscles are practical, as they indeed are, and that it is not so much that we have become accustomed to our twelve eye muscles in the progress of our individual lives, but that the mode of eye movement is not solely the result of a free will directed by specific demands of the sense of sight. On the contrary, its important movements are predetermined by the inborn muscle system.

Given the large variety of applications of the sense of sight, it is also clear that the eye muscles serve many purposes. Thus the way in which the eyes move facilitates or altogether makes possible many aspects of visual perception in ways which we are far from understanding. One might conclude from the many roles to which the eye muscles are adapted that one role or another which one rightly or wrongly holds to be especially important should be selected as the single reason for them, so that the eyes move in one way and not in another. One would then make the same mistake as the old physicians who believed that herbs were created only for use in cures.

It is always useful, however, to consider how the eye would have to move so that this or that which one sees as an important requirement of the sense of sight according to his present knowledge could be achieved as completely as possible. The more one is many-sided in this, the more numerous the points of view one finds from which the true way of moving of the eyes appears as a practical one, and the more principles one constructs from which the method of movement can be teleologically derived, the more fruitful such a method of investigation will be.

In fact, various principles have been perceptively proposed by various researchers in order to derive the rule of the orientation of the eyes. So Meissner, among others, believed that the orientation of both eyes depended upon giving both retinas the mutual position by which as many outside points as possible could be imaged on so-called identical positions. Fick and after him Wundt thought that the line of sight would be so moved and so fixed that in every case the muscles would thereby have the smallest possible stress; later Fick proposed as a leading principle that every position of the line of sight was such that the optic nerve experienced the smallest possible tension. All of these principles as well as two additional ones proposed by Helmholtz will find their substantiation below. Just the number of them indicates that each of them suffers from narrowness. All of them, further, start more or less from the assumption that the newborn is completely free to choose this or that orientation as though the motives which finally determine this choice flow from the appropriate principle. The following section will show that the orientation of the eyes in its principal rules is already indicated in the inborn mechanism of the muscle system, and the newborn is mechanically required to move his eyes at least approximately according to Listing's Law. These principles do not in any way lose their sense, however, for what one saw earlier as chosen in the progress of the individual's life can be interpreted as the inheritance of the lives of countless generations. Further, these principles can be judged as perpetual themes of individual lives from which perhaps small anomalies of the muscle system are corrected and the mode of eye movement is matched to individual requirements.

As little value as I thus give to such more or less teleological considerations, I must nevertheless keep in mind how easily one can thereby confuse origin with purpose, especially in a still inadequately researched area such as the functions of the sense of sight, which is still a contesting ground for diametrically opposed opinions. I will therefore attempt not to try to derive the rules of eye movement *a priori* but rather to show them as consequences of laws already known to us, and from them to derive the advantages which they offer us in the use of the eyes.

It has already been explained that the laws of eye movement which actually apply permit a great simplicity of innervation, and that this is a very great advantage for the easy mastering of eye movements. The next section will discuss further to what degree this law of eye movements must appear as highly practical for purely mechanical reasons. It remains for me here only to discuss the advantages which Listing's Law offers in bringing the retinas into a position beneficial for space perception.

The first advantage is that rolling the eyes about the line of sight is almost completely avoided both with fixed and with moving eyes. The main purpose of our voluntary eye movements is always to see the object of our attention as clearly as possible, in other words, to bring its retinal image to the place of sharpest vision. Rolling the eyes about the line of sight does not aid in reaching this goal. We would see neither better nor more clearly if we rolled the eye about the line of sight and therewith let the retinal image roll about the point of sight.

Such a rolling of the eyes indeed would not only have no purpose, but would make more difficult the grasping of spatial relationships of external objects, because they would destroy the correspondence between the observation of the quiescent and the moving eye. If we fixate a long straight line, it is imaged on a given retinal meridian. From the image of this line we perceive more exactly the part which lies near the point of sight. If we then move our fixation along the line, and its image remains on the same retinal meridian, it is displaced on the retina so to speak along itself, and the single line segments which are sharply perceived one after another will thus always appear to have the same direction. The image would behave otherwise if the eye rolled about the line of sight during the movement of fixation along the line; then the image of the line would always fall on different retinal meridians, and the part of the line presently seen most sharply would correspondingly appear to have a different position than the next following piece, and so forth. In short, the single parts of the line would constantly change their apparent direction and we would believe to see a line whose single parts did not have the same direction and which thus represent a curve. Or at least the line, if we could indeed see it as straight because of its straight retinal image at each moment, would always have to appear to change its position while fixation moved along it, and this apparent rotation would have to occur in the direction opposite to the resulting rotation of the retina about the line of sight.

If we first fixate the point *a* and then want to change fixation to a point *a'* which appears horizontally to the right, we move on the shortest path, that is, we move the gaze in a straight line to the right. This proposed straight line movement of fixation to the right entails a straight line movement of the retinal images a and a' to the left in the case where the eye experiences no cyclorotation. Because we have purposely produced this movement of the retinal image and planned its direction and speed, we do not relate it to a movement of external points as we do when a movement of retinal images occurs without our will. Assuming now, however, that the eye rolls about the line of sight while fixation moves from a to a', then neither a nor a' is displaced in a straight line on the retina, but they describe curved paths. The proposed straight line movement of fixation therefore results in a curved movement of the retinal images rather than the expected straight line displacement. We then relate this to a movement to the degree that the displacement deviates from the planned and expected one.

So we see that any significant cyclorotation during a movement of fixation would lead to a quite different appearance of outward objects for the moving eye than for the quiet one; what appears straight to the steadily fixating eye must appear curved to the moving one, and what appears stationary to one must appear moving to the other and so forth. This unfortunate situation could be resolved only if the cyclorotation were a voluntary one, as is the movement of the line of sight, so that we could master the rotation of the eyes about the line of sight and predict its consequences for the movement of the retinal images, as is possible for us with the movement of the line of sight. In fact, the attempt has been made to master this. But if we wanted to construct such an experiment completely independent of its theoretical improbability, and to forget on the one hand how infinitely more difficult the mastering of eye movements would be and on the other how difficult the perception of space must become, then many facts would still show the incorrectness of this hypothesis proposed by Helmholtz. Some of these facts are discussed in the laws of innervation above and will be proved further below. Also, it will be shown later that in reality each cyclorotation during a fixation movement leads to the sensory confusions just discussed as soon as the rotation exceeds a certain very small size.

We have seen above that Listing's Law of eye movements is characterized in that rolling about the line of sight in the smaller fixation space is almost completely avoided, and is only small even in the peripheral parts of the larger fixation space. I will show later that even the latter is compensated by the associated rotation of the head exactly in those relationships where it could most easily be disturbing. *Listing's Law therefore has the advantage that it brings spatial perception of the moving eye into the greatest possible agreement with the perceptions of fixed eyes, and that the movements of the retinal images are harmonized with the intended fixation movements.* Thus, if we wanted to be teleological we could derive Listing's Law quite directly from the *principle of avoided rolling about the line of sight.* (This principle should not be confused with the principle of orientation given by Helmholtz, which will be discussed in a later section.)

A second advantage of Listing's Law is that with distant vision both eyes are always oriented toward outside objects in nearly equal fashion. It is known that each point of one retina corresponds to a point of the other such that both give the impression of the same direction in outside space and they fortunately lead to an easily fused single image. If these so-called identical or "cover points" were ordered in exactly congruent manner in both retinas, as far as they can be reciprocally placed, then the lines connecting each pair of cover points would lie parallel to one another. But now, as will be thoroughly shown later, the arrangement of cover points is not quite congruent. It always deviates slightly from congruence so that the ideal according to which each distant outward point should be imaged with parallel lines of sight on covering points can be at least adequately approached in the case where the retina is held in the appropriate position. The latter is now fairly well accomplished through Listing's Law, because according to it the two eyes always rotate about parallel axes with distant vision so that each two direction lines belonging to identical positions in both eyes must remain nearly parallel in every position if they are that way in one distant position.

With near objects of sight, the laws of geometrical projection make it entirely impossible that all simultaneously visible outside points can be imaged on cover points of the double retina; rather, one retinal image must generally not be congruent with the other. They cannot fall on entirely identical positions even with an advantageous position of the retinas relative to one another according to the law. The requirement that each outward object should be imaged on covering points, or as one could also say, *the principle of the largest horopter,* thus loses the largest part of its justification with near vision. Furthermore, just this incongruence of the retinal images and their non-identical position helps us in depth perception and in seeing solid bodies, as will be shown later. Similarly, the way in which the eyes move and especially the deviation from Listing's Law which thus occurs in near vision is of advantage for binocular perception. We usually observe near objects with a lowered fixation plane. With such a position of the fixation plane and diverging lines of sight, however, the two horizontal dividing lines according to Listing's Law would be significantly tilted relative to the fixation plane. But in fact, as we see, this is not the case; rather with this fixation position the retinas are positioned so that the horizontal dividing lines nearly always remain close to the fixation plane. This gives, for instance, the advantage in reading that the line being read is imaged in both eyes nearly identically and not doubled with intersecting images, which would have to occur in this orientation according to Listing's Law. In general, the occurrence of double images with a significant difference in height is avoided by the deviation from this law. Such double images, which differ from one another primarily in the lateral direction (which cannot at all be avoided in near vision but concern clear vision much less), help rather to mediate the correct localization of the retinal images in the dimension of depth.

One could teleologically explain deviations from the orientation of Listing's Law from the advantages which the converging double eye obtains from these deviations. They would have no value otherwise because it is understood that the eyes generally move by amounts determined in the interest of vision.

In Chapter 13, *Mechanical prerequisites,* Hering discusses the subject of kinematics, which of course had been extensively treated by Helmholtz and other predecessors. He clearly defines the three-dimensional forces of rotation, the axes of rotation, and starts to discuss such interesting problems in three-dimensional rotations as, for example, the non-commutativity of rotational operations. Hering puts forward infinitesimal rotation as an elegant approach to these problems.

In Chapter 14, *The law of equal retinal position with equal fixation position,* Hering considers Donders' Law. He discusses the experimental fact that cyclorotation is indeed constant within the 'smaller fixation space', and that it changes as a function of vergence. Of special interest is his discussion extending the monocular Donder's Law to treat the double eye. Clearly, binocular application of the monocular Donder's Law approaches closely to what we now call "Hering's Law of equal innervation of corresponding muscles."

Hering next treats the non-willed or involuntary nature of cyclorotations. He concedes that "trick" special movements are possible, like wriggling the ears, but he points out the important observation that voluntary cyclorotations are not used, even when these would be most helpful, as in cases of clinical muscle pareses. Recently, Balliet and Nakayama have demonstrated training of voluntary versional cyclorotations in a few hard-working motivated subjects – their technique involved linear afterimages tracking slowly rotating linear targets.

Hering discusses cyclovergences and shows that these are minimal with cyclodisparities presented as vertical lines. Using his exquisite 'double-line' experiments, he shows that the cyclofusion due to control nervous system computation has such quick dynamics that cyclovergence is quite unlikely to have occurred under his conditions. He next reviews some experiments in which the great Helmholtz erred; this involved misuse of a Dove prism which produced a tilt of vertical lines *and also* some other vertical and horizontal disparities. Hering goes on to describe his own stereoscope; he discusses his positive results for neural computations and his negative results for true cyclovergence eye movements. Of special interest is his discussion of temporary violations of Donder's Law which is similar to the now well-known dynamic violation of Hering's Law (Dynamic and static violations of Hering's Law of Equal Innervation, Bahill, A.T., Ciuffreda, K.J., Kenyon, R.V., and Stark, L. in press, *Am. J. Opt.,* 1976).

In Chapter 15 on *The law of orientation with parallel lines of sight,* Hering takes up Listing's Law. This can be stated geometrically as Listing himself did – that the eye rotates as if about an axis in Listing's plane. A verbal equivalent is that no true cyclorotation can occur with the head fixed.

Three alternate coordinate systems are used in discussing kinematics of the eye. For many purposes Listing's Coordinate System has advantages; it utilizes meridian, eccentricity and cyclorotation (m, e, C_L). Helmholtz's coordinate system employs elevation, azimuth and cyclorotation (l, z, C_H); and Fick's coordinate system uses longitude, latitude and cyclorotation (g, t, C_F). In general $C_L \neq C_H \neq C_F$. With Listing's coordinate system, C_L equals true, physical cyclorotation.

According to Listing's Law $C_L = 0$. Therefore, in the region where Listing's Law is valid, C_H will have real values as a function of elevation and azimuth, $C_H = f(l, z)$. These are tabulated by Helmholtz, and Hering reproduces the table here (Table 1). Table 1 thus gives the values of C_H, cyclorotation in Helmholtz' coordinate system for which no true cyclorotation occurs, $C_L = 0$, and equivalently for which the eyeball rotates according to Listing's Law. These are also experimentally found values that thus demonstrate the validity of Listing's Law.

Hering discusses the need for an operational definition of primary position and shows how horizontal and vertical movements that show no false torsion have as their intersection the primary position. He then discusses Listing's Plane as the collection of axes of rotation for horizontal and vertical eye movements and oblique eye movements within the narrow or smaller fixation space. Listing's Plane is, of course, the plane through the center of rotation perpendicular to the line of sight.

Hering's great attention to careful detailed control of his experimental techniques is especially well demonstrated in this chapter. He points out that in using afterimages it is not sufficient to use an afterimage parallel to the meridian of rotation or one perpendicular to it, but it is necessary to use both (in the form of a cross). Hering points out that "if one wants to gain information about the orientation of the retina from the apparent rotation of the afterimage, one must pay attention to how and to what extent the altered form and position of the retinal image depends on the external objects on which the afterimage appears, and with whose lines and contours the position of the afterimage will be compared."

I experienced this in a dramatic way while staying in an old Japanese inn. I had an oblique view of a paper wall with a sharp wooden rectangular mesh through which early morning sunlight was diffusing. If I closed my eyes but kept the oblique fixation constant, the afterimage appeared rectangular. When, however, I rotated my eyes to a blank wall with approximate straight-ahead gaze, the afterimage appeared to be very distorted; the rectangles now formed acute and obtuse angles. Thus, in this simple experiment it was clear that eye movement produced a change in interpretation of a constant retinal afterimage. The normal compensatory mechanism which caused an oblique image and afterimage to appear rectangular during the direct visual experience (and during interpretation of the afterimage while the closed eyes continued stationary) was not utilized when the closed eyes were in approximately straight-ahead position. Now the oblique pattern appeared as it was in the afterimage on the retina. Thus the compensatory mechanism was informed of eye position by corollary discharge or efferent copy.

Hering discusses four interesting experiments. First, afterimages remain parallel to calibrating threads on making *cardinal* movements from the primary position. This is also true when making 45° oblique movements if, and only if, the afterimages are parallel or perpendicular to the oblique line of rotation. In a second experiment, after tilting the head but on keeping the line of sight fixed with respect to the wall, the afterimages are observed to rotate. This, of course, is because the eyeball is in a changed position with respect to the orbit even though it is fixed with respect to the threads on the wall. In an elegant third experiment, Hering demonstrates the false torsion phenomena. Here the afterimage is arranged to be a cross in parallel and perpendicular position to the oblique meridian of rotation. The cross which originally had two orthogonal arms now appears nonrectangular and oblique. Helmholtz, of course, had previously done this experiment but with only single vertical or single horizontal afterimages. It was thus possible to interpret the rotation as possibly due to a cyclorotation of the eyeball. When, however, Hering uses the orthogonal cross and the two arms of the cross rotate in *opposite* directions, it is clear that false torsion is not at all involved with true cyclorotation. No change of the cross is seen, of course, in making cardinal movements. In a fourth experiment, Hering arranges the cross to be perpendicular and parallel to the meridian of rotation and demonstrates that no false torsion occurs.

In Chapter 16, *Determination of retinal position with afterimages,* Hering conducts another set of very careful experiments in this difficult area of physiological optics. He develops a frame with threads in several colors and a bitebar which enables him to rotate the head about the line of sight. He takes special pains to make certain that the lines of sight of the two eyes are parallel. He also uses a mirror technique to help in precise adjustment of the subject. Hering states, "The apparatus appears complicated but when it is once calibrated saves much time and effort, for one can use it for the most varied experiments in which it is useful to exactly control eye position and to know the absolute position of the point of rotation." It is extraordinary that with his experimental excellence so well demonstrated, people have still mistakenly taken Hering to be an 'armchair' physiologist.

He now goes through careful experimental definition of the primary position as that point from which cardinal movements without apparent rotation of afterimages can be performed. Hering then reviews some of the current literature and shows that while Helmholtz made an error because he did not control the nodding of the head in his apparatus, on the contrary Berthold seemed to have performed these experiments more correctly. Hering feels that he can assert Listing's Law to be experimentally valid to within plus or minus a degree while within the smaller bifixation space.

In Chapter 17, *Determination of retinal position with binocular images,* Hering describes extensions of his apparatus so that he can rotate four threads, two of which are binocularly fused and two of which are seen monocularly. He then is able to test for parallel lines of sight of the two eyes. Deviations from Listing's Law occur in that considerable cyclovergence is produced (i) as a function of horizontal vergence, (ii) secondary to vestibular action, and (iii) especially with head-nod in the forward direction. At this point, Hering discusses the individual variations of the different illustrative and illustrious subjects that had so far reported their results – Helmholtz, Hering and Berthold.

In Chapter 18, *Investigation of retinal position with converging lines of sight,* Hering still further extends his apparatus so as to be certain he has both a horizontal visual plane and a vertical observation plane. By this time the experiments in which he was the sole subject were straining him and his motivation is sorely tested, – "In general, one can investigate the orientation of the retinas at near positions with the afterimage method and must only experiment binocularly with them so that the afterimage is elicited in just one eye, while the fixation point with near vision would be visible with both eyes. I had already begun these experiments once, but had had to give them up at that time because my eyes were already very strained by much experimentation. It is especially difficult to keep the afterimage alive with strong convergence of the lines of sight because each large muscular effort of the eyes weakens the afterimage. Very intensive afterimages are therefore necessary for these experiments. At present I am not in a condition to take up these experiments again because my eyes have many demands on them from other investigations."

With his (tired!) eye, Hering now investigates the monocular Listing's Law and shows that it is not true with convergence. By comparison with Helmholtz's table (Table 2) for C_H as a function of angle of gaze when $C_L = 0$, he can show that the deviation for experimentally determined C_H from C_H for Listing's Law means that the eye has actually cyclorotated. This provides an opportunity for him to develop the difference between empiricism and nativism. Empiricism suggests that the deviation occurs in order to obtain clear vision and has been developed by practice; nativism suggests that the deviation has no reason but is an inborn mechanism. There could be only one innervation for near vision, and subsequent changes, for example in vertical fixation, add to the mechanical force output of the muscles, thus producing true cyclorotations and violations of Listing's Law.

With binocular viewing, Hering shows agreement with Helmholtz in that convergence and downward vertical rotation both produce cyclodivergence rotation. With an occluder blocking *binocular disparity* or 'opening the loop' of the binocular disparity-vergence system or with far vision, cycloconvergence is produced. In a further beautiful set of experiments, Hering shows that accommodation producing accommodative convergence (in the covered eye) yields cyclodivergence in the seeing eye. He then develops the theory which these experiments support – the innervation for near vision goes not only to accommodation and to the adductor muscles but also to the other muslces in a not yet specified pattern.

It appears that a generalized Donders' Law could be formulated. Donders only stated his law for the monocular case, when both eyes were looking at a distant fixation point and thus had parallel lines of sight. There is a further interesting relationship between Donders' Law, generalized for binocular and near vision, and Hering's Laws themselves. This will be treated more fully in Part IV and in the summary.

Hering indicates that practice appears to have a small effect on the ACA ratio. Whether this is truly valid and what the underlying mechanisms are, is not relevant here. What is important is that it shows that Hering never did deny the possibility of experience, practice, and learning overlaying or having a supplementary effect on basic inborn mechanisms.

In Chapter 19, *On the optical meaning of the orientation laws,* Hering states the importance of eye movements in the service of vision, "it is clear that the motor apparatus of the visual organ must match its sensory apparatus as the shell does the egg," and makes clear the difference between teleology and the evolutionary mechanisms which underly animal and human physiological mechanisms. Hering is most interested not to confuse the origins of a mechanism and its purpose. He discusses the multi-functional aspects of the eye movements and purposes put forward by others – Meissner, Fick, Wundt and Helmholtz.

It is important to clarify that although nativism vs. empiricism seems to have birth as the dividing line, the situation is somewhat more complicated. Innate mechanisms should also include mechanisms that unfold in development; for example, reading readiness in children may be a result of neurological developmental mechanisms unrelated to school or other experiences. In general, innate mechanisms are genetic and selected through evolution. Similarly, included under empiricism would be learning both *before* and after birth. For example, reflexes in the embryo may go on *in utero* for several months and may influence development of the nervous system. Empiricism is concerned with that mapping of the world onto the central nervous system which reoccurs for each generation; nativism stresses the mapping of the world onto the central nervous system through evolutionary selection of the appropriate genetic-memory mechanisms.

Hering himself suggests that simplicity of innervation is the guiding principle for the control of eye movements. He postpones the discussion of mechanical reasons to Part III, and proceeds to discuss the causes and consequences for *vision* of these orientation control laws. Listing's Law, he says, is appropriate for spatial perception in monocular viewing. When we observe a straight line either in a stationary fashion or by moving the fovea along the straight line, it can appear straight statically as well as dynamically only if Listing's Law of no cyclorotation is obeyed; otherwise it would appear curved or changed in orientation on dynamic viewing.

For binocular vision, the orientation laws maximize corresponding points in far vision. Unfortunately, they cannot also be congruent for near vision, but can at least minimize the discrepancies utilizing the principle of 'the largest horopter.' This is also true for the secondary deviations and the associated tilt in convergence when reading. Listing's Law, however, helps to keep the horizontal dividing lines in the fixation plane and aids both depth perception and minimization of double images.

Now Hering turns to Helmholtz' important frame-of-reference computation associated with voluntary movements. (This is now known to be true only for saccadic eye movements, whether voluntary or not.) He points out the difficulty in carrying out Helmholtz' hypothesis of cyclorotation and as well the complex computations that would be necessary to take this latter into account.

It is interesting that only ten years after the publication of Darwin's revolutionary text on evolution, Hering clearly interprets the inborn orientation laws of human eye movements in terms of evolutionary selection. First, Hering discusses motor and sensory correlation, "Whether one assumes that both are arranged according to a wise plan, or that they have developed with one another and through one another in naturally necessary ways through the animal series, in any case the capabilities of one must bespeak the demands of the other. It follows that the eye muscles are practical, as they indeed are, and that it is not so much that we have become accustomed to our twelve eye muscles in the progress of our individual lives, but that the mode of eye movement is not solely the result of a free will directed by specific demands of the sense of sight. On the contrary, its important movements are predetermined by the inborn muscle system." And then a little later in leading us on to Part III, *On the Eye Muscles,* he states, "The following section will show that the orientation of the eyes in its principal rules is already indicated in the inborn mechanism of the muscle system, and the newborn is mechanically required to move his eyes at least approximately according to Listing's Law. These principles do not in any way lose their sense, however, for what one saw earlier as chosen in the progress of the individual's life can be interpreted as the inheritance of the lives of countless generations."

20. *Background about the Eye Muscles*

Although an investigation of the mechanisms of the single muscles does not really belong in the plan of this work, but rather in the physiology of the single eye, I find it necessary to dedicate a special chapter to it to illustrate that the mechanisms of the eye musculature also permit the derivation of several grounds for the correctness of the laws of innervation given above.

For an exact treatment of the problem of eye movement it has recently become customary to think of the muscles as substituted by infinitely thin elastic threads or elastic lines. These are fastened to the orbit at one end and to the eyeball at the other in the geometric center of the insertion lines, which are known to be fairly broad but are otherwise completely isolated. Such a thread, if its tension were analogous to that of the true muscles, would always have the goal of shortening itself in order to come into the condition of balance of its elastic forces. To this end it would always take the position which gave it the smallest possible length under the governing conditions. But this is the case only when its entire length lies in a plane which also goes through the fixed rotation point of the sphere. This includes not only the part of the thread which runs in a straight line through the orbit but also the part which lies on the eyeball (which can be thought of as a sphere). This is also the plane in which the elastic thread attempts to move the line of sight, and the diameter of the eyeball perpendicular to this plane would be the axis about which it exerted rotational force.

The position of the ocular insertion of an eye muscle changes relative to its orbital insertion with every change of position of the eyeball. If one now considers the muscles in the manner discussed as elastic lines with single point insertions, then the changed positions of their ocular origin points generally result in a changed positions of their planes of movement and of their half axes of rotational force. Only when the thread has not left its original movement plane during the change of position of the eyeball does the half axis of its rotational force remain unchanged.

This analysis of the imagined elastic threads cannot be applied without reservation to the true muscles; as often happens, the relationships are quite different. The eye muscles are fastened to the eyeball with very broad insertions, so that when the eyeball rotates the individual portions of the insertion line of the muscle change positions in quite varied ways. When the eye is rotated upward out of the primary position about a horizontal axis, for instance, the lower tendons of the lateral and medial recti are lengthened and the upper ones shortened. The first thus are more strongly stressed, their tension increases, and that of the upper one contrastingly decreases. The result, as Helmholtz (11) has already noted, is that the path resulting from the tensions on its single elements moves nearer to the lower, more strongly stressed elements, and thus no longer lies in the middle of the muscle. So it happens that the pulling direction and the half axis of rotational force of this muscle are not significantly displaced in spite of raising or sinking of the eye, as would be the case if the muscle were only an elastic thread inserted at a single point. From this we can also conclude that the muscles do not slide so freely on the eyeball and cannot move in the orbital cavity as freely as would be assumed with the elastic threads.

All of those calculations of the axes of rotational force of the single muscles with various positions of the eyes which are made on the basis of the inadequate assumption just discussed thus cannot give realistic results, even if we do not consider all other possible sources of error in such calculations.

In order to determine the ocular and orbital insertions of the eye muscles, Reute fixed the swelled eyeball in the orbit such that it was approximately in the position referred to above as the primary position and then considered the insertion point to be the geometric center of each single insertion line or surface. His method should have given approximately correct results, and I will thus base the following on his data and also assume that the investigated eye was in the primary position. Because the pulling direction which results from the sum of the fibres of the rectus muscles does not change significantly with small displacements of the eyeball, as I have just shown, the approximate errors of that assumption are not important in any case.

A plane through the two insertion points determined in the manner given, and through the rotation point of the eye, might be called the *muscle plane*. The half axis about which the muscle exerts rotational force on the eye is then perpendicular to this plane at the center of rotation, if the muscle is truly fixed only on its orbital end and is not for instance hindered by other sideward connections in the orbit. It will be positioned in the orbit as the possibilities of its elasticity determine, as though it were freely suspended between the orbital wall and the bulb. Reute assumes the latter, and this assumption cannot entail any significant error at least for the primary position. The half axis about which one muscle attempts to rotate the eye at primary position will be indicated below as the *primary half axis* of this muscle.

From Reute's measurements one can only conclude that in the primary position each two so-called antagonists of the eye attempt to rotate about nearly one and the same axis in opposite directions, and that the common primary axis of the medial and lateral recti is perpendicular to the horizontal plane through the point of rotation of the eye, while the common axis of the superior and inferior recti and the common primary axis of the obliques lie in this horizontal plane itself. The first has an angle of about 19° and the latter an angle of about 52° with the line connecting the rotation points of the eyes. Figure 24 illustrates the position of these axes for the left eye; *bb* is the baseline, *gg* the line of sight running through the point of rotation, *m* the point of rotation, *m-ri* the primary half axis of the inferior rectus, *m-rs* that of the superior rectus, *m-oi* that of the inferior oblique, and *m-os* that of the superior oblique. One can think of the primary half axis of the medial rectus as standing perpendicular to the plane of the paper at *m*, above the paper, and that of the lateral rectus in like manner below the paper.

Consider a horizontal plane located at the primary position through the common axis of the two obliques, and through the common axis of the superior and inferior recti. Further imagine two vertical planes through the common axis of the medial and lateral recti such that one also goes through the axis of the two obliques and the other also through the axis of the superior and inferior recti. In this way the eyeball will be divided by these three planes into eight parts or sectors. Each of these sectors has exactly three edges, each

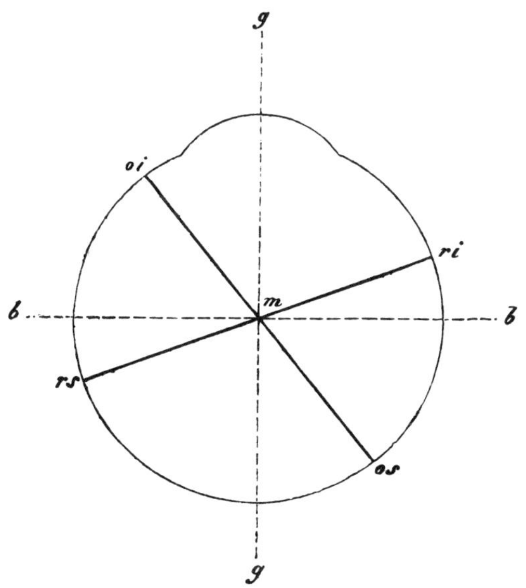

Fig. 24.

of which coincides with the primary half axis of one of the six muscles. It can now be determined which muscles must be innervated in order to elicit a rotational force about a given half axis. One apparently has only to consider in which of the eight sectors the given half axis lies; the three muscles whose half axes are the three edges of this sector must work together to elicit the demanded rotation. According to the rule of the parallelepiped described above and the moment of rotation, the relationship of the three forces can be found with which the three muscles must engage the eyeball for the given purpose (Fick (7)). Each of the eight sectors is further bordered by three plane surfaces; if the given half axis falls on one of these surfaces, then the two muscles whose half axes constitute the straight sides of these surfaces work together to elicit the demanded rotation, and the force relationship necessary for this is determined according to the parallelogram of the moments of rotation. Finally, if the given half axis coincides from the beginning with one of the six muscle half axes, that is naturally the muscle whose sole contraction can elicit the demanded rotation without further ado.

The musculature of the eyeball is thus so arranged that at the primary position a rotation about any given half axis can be elicited with three muscles, and in special cases only one or two muscles must be active. If the eyeball is brought from its primary position into any other position, then the muscle half axes will also have changed their positions more or less because their ocular insertions have deviated with respect to the orbit. But as before we will always be able to consider the six muscle half axes as edges of eight sectors of the eyeball even though the form (Gestalt) of the latter will have changed somewhat. What we have just said about the primary position will also apply as before.

Given that it can occur that the six eye muscles are not innervated at all, the eye will assume a certain equilibrium position which one can indicate as the resting position. We do not know exactly which position that is; it is indeed not known to us whether the case of a complete cessation of all innervation of the eye muscles can occur at all in a state of health. Several experiences make it indeed not unlikely that all the eye muscles are more or less innervated during vision, that they therefore possess a certain constant tonus dependent on innervation, and that there is therefore no position of the seeing eye in which it finds itself only under the influence of the independent elastic tensions of the eye muscles.

Like any other muscles, the eye muscles are so mounted at their ends that they are always in a certain state of tension, with the consequence that even when they are not innervated at all they attempt to shorten and to pull the eye each according to its direction. In the absence of all innervation, the eye in its resting position would remain still not because there is no pull exercised on it but because the moments of rotation of the six muscles oppose each other so that no rotation results. In general, whenever the eye stands still in any position the resulting moment of all six moments of rotation of the six muscles is equal to zero. The moment resulting from the moments of rotation of any five muscles is just as large as the moment of rotation of the sixth, with the latter diametrically opposed; the moment resulting from any four muscles is equal to but opposite from that of the two remaining moments of rotation, and so forth. If one muscle were completely cut through while the eye was in the hypothetical resting position, then a moment of rotation resulting from the tension of the other five muscles would immediately apply, and the eye would experience a rotation although no innervation had occurred; conversely, if a muscle is innervated and contracts while the eye is in the resting position, then its moment of rotation would grow, thus exceeding the diametrically opposed pulls of the five other muscles and their resulting moments of rotation, and consequently would lead to a rotation of the eyeball.

The half axis about which this rotation occurs does not depend only on the position of the moment of rotation of the current muscle; *that is, the half axis of rotational force of one muscle is not necessarily the half axis of the true rotation which it elicits.* Just as the direction which a ship moves forward depends not only on the direction of the applied force, but also on the direction of the resistances of the rudder or the current, for instance, so also the resistances which oppose a rotation of the eyeball help to determine the direction of rotation, that is, the position of the half axis about which it occurs. The resistances which come into consideration in an eye rotation lie partly in those muscles which are activated, partly in those which also connect with the orbital wall, and partly in the unavoidable friction. Concerning the resistances which are not based on the musculature, at least as long as the line of sight moves in the middle part of fixation space according to Listing's Law we can assume without significant error that they always work in a direction diametrically opposed to the rotation. Thus they can impede but not change the direction of rotation. It is different with the resistances which the activated muscles offer.

The rotation of the eyeball begins as soon as one muscle is innervated and its moment of rotation is increased by a certain amount. We now assume that the increase in power occurring in the muscle is adequate only for an infinitely small rotation, and consider that this rotation truly occurs about that half axis on which the moment of rotation of the active muscle lay before the beginning of the rotation. Through the infinitely small rotation the insertions of the eye muscles on the bulb will be displaced infinitely little relative to their insertions on the orbit, whereby some of the five inactive muscles become infinitesimally longer and others perhaps shorter. The former will now have stronger tension and the latter weaker; the moments of rotation of the former will have grown and those of the latter decreased. In addition, the half axes of their rotational forces can change position infinitesimally by displacement of the muscle insertions. The moment of rotation resulting from the five inactive muscles can thus change its position infinitesimally, so that in the course of the infinitesimal rotation it does not remain diametrically opposed to the moment of rotation of the active muscle. Thus while the active muscle attempts to rotate the eye about its half axis, the five other muscles attempt to rotate not about the opposite half axis but about another half axis. *From this double rotational force resulting from the active muscle on one side and the resistances on the other side, one finds that rotational force which the eyeball follows.*

Consequently it cannot be asserted, as has happened frequently, that under all circumstances a muscle can at least begin a rotation about the half axis of its moment of rotation. For the moment of rotation resulting from the five inactive muscles need not change its position only *after* the beginning, but can already change it *with* the beginning of the rotation. Only when the resistances which oppose a rotation are so ordered that their resulting moment remains diametrically opposed to the moment of the active muscles even during the movement can the rotation truly occur about the half axis of the active muscle, whether the rotation is infinitely small or of finite size.

The resistances which the pulling force of a muscle encounters are less important if the moment which the active muscle elicits is very large in comparison to the resistances. But this is not the case; usually, the moment of rotation of the active muscle only slightly exceeds the moment resulting from the sum of the resistances, and especially the resulting moment of the remaining muscles. Otherwise the eyeball would not always show the same security of movement which we perceive for it, but would be thrown about repeatedly, as is the case with cramps of the eye muscles. For this reason it is a mistake to neglect the resistances of the muscles not especially innervated in an eye movement, and to take no note of the way in which the eye muscles reciprocally control one another. One often speaks of the activities of a single eye muscle as though the five others were not there at all, as though with each innervation of one muscle the moment resulting from the five others were not almost as large as the moment of the innervated muscle, and as though the position of the axis of rotation were not therefore of the greatest influence.

In the following table Reute (26) has summarized the coordinates of the ocular and orbital insertions of the eye muscles for the eye position given above. The origin point of the coordinates is the middle point of the eye, though this may not coincide with the point of rotation. The axis of *x* coincides with the horizontal diameter perpendicular to the visual axis, the axis of *y* with the visual axis, and the axis *z* with the vertical diameter. The direction of positive *x* goes outward, the direction of positive *y* goes backward, and that of positive *z* goes upward.

Figure 25 shows the vertical projection of the six muscles on the horizontal plane which goes through the middle point of the eye, according to measurements made by Reute.

Table 5

	Insertions			Origins		
	x	y	z	x	y	z
Superior Rectus	+ 2,00mm	–5,667	+10	–10,67	+32	+4
Inferior Rectus	+ 2,20mm	–5,767	–10	–10,8	+32	–4
Lateral Rectus	+10,80mm	–5,00	0	– 5,4	+ 32	0
Medial Rectus	– 9,90mm	6,00	0	–14,67	+ 32	0
Superior Oblique Tendon	+ 2,00mm	+3,00	+ 11	–14,1	–10	+12
Inferior Oblique	+ 8,00mm	+6,00	0	– 8,1	– 6	–15

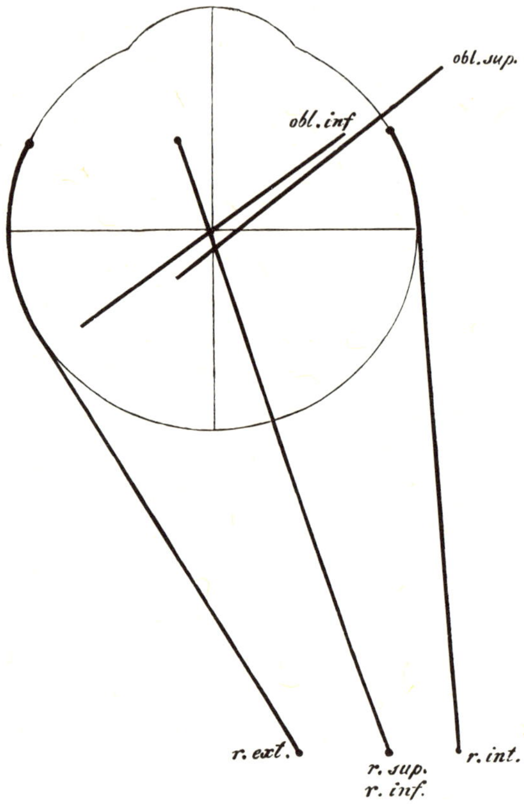

Fig. 25.

21. *On the Single Actions of the Eye Muscles*

A muscle can truly turn the eye only on the axis about which it exerts rotational force if no resistances oppose this rotation, or only if such resistances exactly oppose the direction of the muscle pull. Under such circumstances only the lateral and medial recti move the line of sight in straight lines, but all other muscles move it in curved paths, and specifically the medial rectus directly inward, the lateral rectus directly outward, the superior rectus upward and inward, the inferior rectus downward and inward, the superior oblique downward and outward, and the inferior oblique upward and outward. In figure 26 I have indicated the path which the lines of sight would describe on a plane perpendicular to them in the primary position. The position of the axes of rotation is assumed as given above. The separation between the rotation point of the eye and the vertical plane is taken to be the line *dd*. At the end of each path I have also shown with a darker line the apparent position which an originally horizontal afterimage would assume at the corresponding place on the line of sight, that is, an afterimage which the eye received from a horizontal stripe in primary position. The length of each path corresponds to a rotation of the eye of 50° about the corresponding half axis. Each numbered mark on each path shows how much the line of sight is shifted after the angle of rotation increases by 10°. One sees that the line of sight shifts the most slowly with rotations about the primary half axes of the oblique muscles, and at the same time the position of the afterimage at the end of the path shows that the rolling of the eyes about the line of sight is very important here; the curved path of the latter is hyperbolic. With the same angle of rotation the line of sight describes a longer and also hyperbolic path when the rotation occurs about the primary half axes of the superior or inferior recti. At the same time, the rolling of the line of sight is smaller. The longest and indeed straight path, without an accompanying rolling about the line of sight, is described by rotation of the lateral or medial recti about the primary half axis.

But in fact, the resistances which each rotation of the eye encounters are not always exactly opposed to the pulling direction of the active muscle. We will next investigate how these resistances relate to one another when only one muscle is contracted. For the reasons given above we consider the resistances lying outside the muscles to always oppose the direction of pulling.

The contraction of the medial rectus will find its main resistance in the lateral rectus because this is the one which thereby is especially stretched; in the same way the medial rectus determines the main resistance in the contraction of the lateral rectus. Both muscles indeed attempt to turn the eye on the same axis in opposite direc-

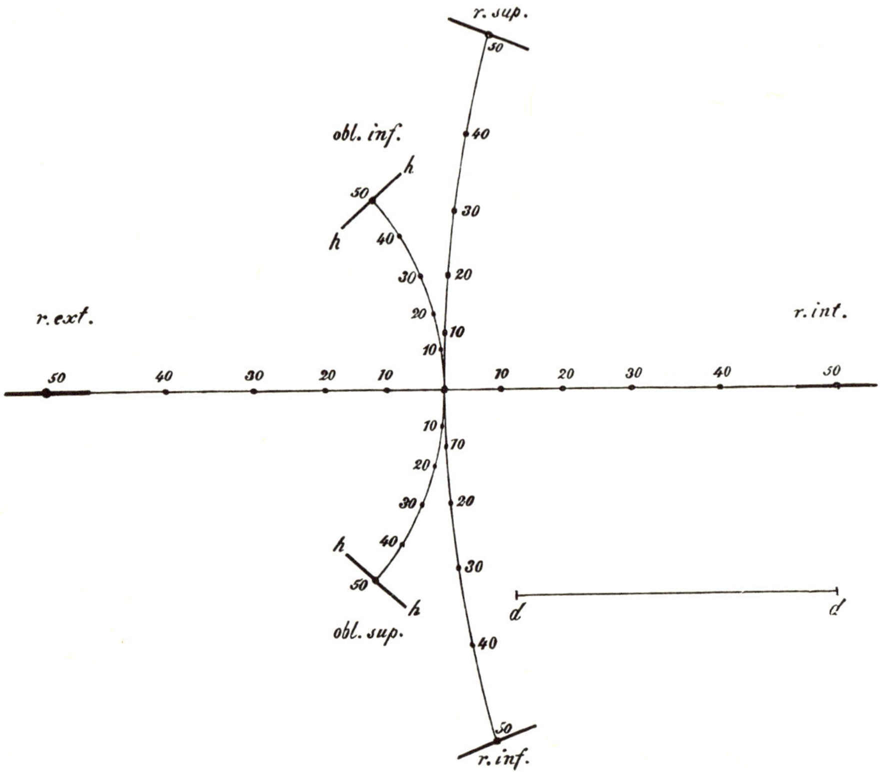

Fig. 26.

tions. The resistance of the lateral rectus will therefore limit the rotational force of the medial rectus about the horizontal axis, but cannot pull it out of its path; the same applies in reverse for the medial rectus with respect to the lateral rectus. To date no reason has been given that the rotation should not truly occur about the vertical axis in both cases. We will now see how the other four muscles behave.

The pulling directions of the superior and inferior recti will not be significantly changed when the eye is turned inward or outward. Because the tension on one remains as large as that on the other they both maintain equilibrium during the movement as before, and can therefore have no disturbing influence on the direction of movement. One could only consider that they might assist in large rotations of the eye inward, because their two moments of rotation are then no longer diametrically opposed but can give a small resulting moment.

Analogously, the two obliques are perhaps stretched somewhat with rotation inward and are pulled upon somewhat less with rotation outward. In the case of inward movement, the loop which this pair of muscles so to say forms around the eyeball lies somewhat behind the largest circle which they spanned in the primary position. In outward movement they lie somewhat in front of this position. This will have no other results for the rotation referred to than to inhibit it somewhat inward and to enhance it somewhat outward. These muscles too will have no significant influence on the direction of rotation. The result is thus *that both the lateral rectus and the medial rectus, in spite of the resistances present, are able to rotate the eye from primary position nearly about the axis about which they attempt to rotate it.*

But the other four muscles behave quite differently. If one of these contracted alone, which indeed is not normally the case in reality, then the eye would in no way be able to rotate on that axis about which the rotational force acts in the primary position, and the line of sight would describe a quite different plane than that indicated in figure 26 for the case of rotation without resistances.

For example, if the superior rectus began to contract alone its principal resistance would be in the antagonistic inferior rectus, which would be stretched, but because it exactly opposes the superior rectus it could only reduce the rotational force and not deviate the movement from its path. Aside from the inferior rectus, the superior oblique would also offer a significant resistance because its ocular insertion must move away from the trochlea if the eye is to be rotated upward about the primary half axis of the superior oblique. The inferior oblique does not have a correspondingly stronger tension but instead becomes somewhat relaxed. The rotational force of the superior oblique, which is increased by the activation, no longer finds the necessary resistance on the side of the inferior oblique and will therefore be revealed because it too turns the eye when the superior oblique rotates it. So it will happen that the rotation occurs about quite different axes than the primary half axis of the superior rectus, and it is especially apparent that a strong rolling of the eyes about the line of sight would occur and the latter would be less raised than would be the case without the resistance of the superior oblique. Of course the axes about which the rotation would truly occur cannot be given exactly; but because the other resistances come into play relatively much less than those of the inferior rectus and the superior obliques it is clear *that with general contraction of the superior rectus the raising of the eye would be accompanied by a rolling about the line of sight so strong that it would never be normally observed in reality.* From this it follows directly *that the sole contraction of this muscle does not occur.*

A quite analogous argument can be made for the inferior rectus, whose sole contraction would find its principle resistance in the superior rectus and the inferior oblique, which by its resistance would similarly permit a strong rolling of the eyes. But because this is not experienced, *the sole contraction of the inferior rectus also cannot be assumed under normal circumstances.* We will see later that this can be observed in pathological cases during paralysis of the superior oblique, a muscle which is normally always associated with the inferior rectus. One can then also prove that the strong rollings which are expected from the theory truly occur. These rollings are therefore principally the result of the resistance which the inferior oblique opposes to the rotational force of the inferior rectus, and are not a result of the inferior rectus attempting to strongly cyclorotate the eye.

Finally, the case of sole contraction of the superior or inferior oblique is to be discussed. Each of these muscles finds its principal resistance in the other as its antagonist. In addition, the superior oblique, which attempts to rotate the line of sight with strong rolling of the eye downward and outward, is opposed by a not insignificant resistance from the superior rectus and medial rectus, as is the inferior oblique by the inferior rectus and the medial rectus. *But because the sole contraction of these muscles normally never occurs, it follows directly that the relatively small movements of the line of sight which they would induce would have to be accompanied by a rolling of the eyes so great that it is never even approximately observed.*

To give an overview of the resistances which each single muscle would encounter with sole contraction of the other muscles, I have in the following placed the active muscle opposite the one which principally opposes its rotational forces. Specifically, they are in the order in which the magnitudes of their resistances come into consideration:

the medial rectus opposes the lateral rectus,
the lateral rectus opposes the medial rectus,
the superior rectus opposes the inferior rectus,
  superior oblique,
the inferior rectus opposes the superior rectus,
  inferior oblique,
the superior oblique opposes the inferior oblique,
  superior rectus, medial rectus,

the inferior oblique opposes the superior oblique,
inferior rectus, medial rectus.

As soon as an oblique participates in one of these muscle combinations either as an active or passive resisting muscle, the movement of the line of sight will be accompanied by a rolling of the eyes about the line of sight stronger than will occur according to Listing's Law, and therefore the lateral rectus and medial rectus are the only eye muscles which can come into isolated use.

When the eye is in its primary position, according to our assumption, the six eye muscles grasp the eyeball such that each two of them are almost exactly antagonists. From this it follows immediatly that the force with which each of the muscles attempts to rotate the eye with its tension is just as large as the diametrically opposing force of its antagonist, and that the rotational force of each muscle is cancelled only by the tension of its antagonist. The moment resulting from the tension on the two antagonistic muscles is therefore zero in the primary position, and if one could suddenly and simultaneously cut through the other four muscles, the eyeball would not noticeably change its position. This is no longer the case in certain secondary positions. If the eye is moved strongly upward from the primary position, for instance, then the medial rectus and the lateral rectus are still nearly but no longer exactly antagonistic; the result is that their two moments of rotation do not completely cancel but that a very small moment of rotation probably results from them. This consists of an upward rolling of the eye, and therefore assists the moment resulting from the combined tension of the two raisers.

From the exact, or at least very near antagonism of each two muscles in the primary position, it further follows that *if the eye is to be moved from the primary position about any axis, the choice of the muscles to be used is not free, but the movement in question is always accomplished with a single kind of innervation and corresponding muscle action. A true vicarious choice among various muscles is therefore not possible for a rotation out of the primary position.*

I want to emphasize this because the opposite opinion is repeatedly voiced by physiologists and opthalmologists. It has been said that four eye muscles would be enough to elicit a rotational force about any half axis. Here there would be only a single muscle combination for each given half axis, which could accomplish rotational forces about this half axis. But because six muscles grasp the eyeball, there are more muscles than are necessary for accomplishing all conceivable movements, and one and the same moment of rotation could thus be elicited with various muscle combinations. Against this, note that if four muscles were adequate for accomplishing every desired moment of rotation, the half axes of their rotational forces would have to lie so that no three fell in the same plane, and that therefore no two muscles could be pure antagonists. But now both are clearly the case in the eye, and for the primary position we can assume pure antagonism of each two muscles without significant error. With this arrangement we can let three planes go through the eyeball, each containing four of the six muscle half axes. This applies exactly only at the primary position and under the assumptions we have made, but even with other eye positions and with somewhat different assumptions each pair of eye muscles remains at least very nearly antagonistic. One could then discuss various combinations of muscles for eliciting one and the same moment only under the assumption that two such antagonists are simultaneously innervated. From the simultaneous tension of two nearly antagonistic muscles, however, only a very small moment would result even with the strongest innervation, and it should not be thought that this highly ineffective way of eliciting a movement would normally occur. The problem is, in fact, much easier for us than it appears to be according to those who think that one and the same movement could be accomplished with varying participations of the muscles.

From Listing's Law we know the axes about which the eye rotates for every given movement. It remains to seek the muscles participating in each of these rotations, and thereby to prove the correctness of the general laws of innervation given earlier. For each rotation with a known half axis, it has been satisfactory to use the rules given above to determine the muscles which can elicit a moment of rotation about the relevant half axis if one implicitly assumes that these muscles are also able to execute the rotation about the given half axis. But we must not limit ourselves to this; we must also include in our calculations the resistances which oppose the rotation in question. The necessary attention to the resistances will of course extraordinarily complicate the consideration in cases where the fortunate circumstance that the six muscles can be understood as three antagonistic pairs does not occur. This holds most rigorously for the primary position. For example, if any half axis is given about which a rotation is possible according to Listing's Law, and we determine the muscles which can elicit a moment of rotation about this half axis, then we generally find *that these are always exactly the antagonists of those muscles which provide the significant resistance to rotation about this half axis.* The resistances of these muscles therefore are more or less exactly diametrically opposed to the rotational force elicited by their antagonists, and therefore cannot significantly deviate the rotation created by the active muscles. As I have mentioned, this applies most exactly at the primary position, and we may therefore neglect for now the muscles which rotate the eye out of this position according to Listing's Law when we determine the resistances.

If we now seek the muscles which move the eye out of the primary position, there is always only one answer for each given

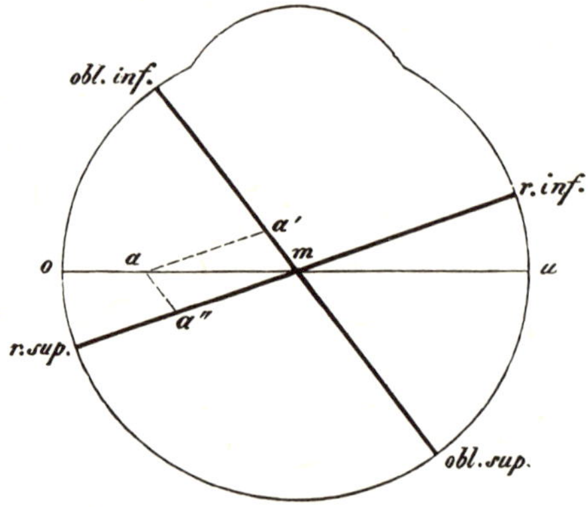

Fig. 27.

direction of movement. As we have seen, all axes which are relevant here lie in the plane vertical to the line of sight, that is in the primary axis plane. For inward rotation from the primary position only the medial rectus can therefore serve, and for outward rotation only the lateral rectus, because their moments of rotation lie in the vertical axis of the primary axis plane. For rotation upward the combined action of the superior rectus and the inferior oblique is necessary, and for downward rotation the combined action of the inferior rectus and the superior oblique. Figure 27 is a horizontal section of the left eye in the primary position. According to Listing's Law, *mo* is the half axis about which the eye must begin a rotation upward and *mu* is the half axis about which a rotation downward must begin. The other radii given in the figure are the half axes of the two obliques and the superior and inferior recti, each labelled with the name of the corresponding muscle. To begin a rotation upward, a moment of rotation on the half axis *mo* must be elicited. This is labeled *ma*. As the figure shows, this moment of rotation can be obtained only by simultaneous innervation of the superior rectus and the inferior oblique such that the former elicits the moment of rotation *ma''*. From these two moments the desired moment of rotation *ma* results. *No other muscle combination is able to elicit this moment of rotation ma.*

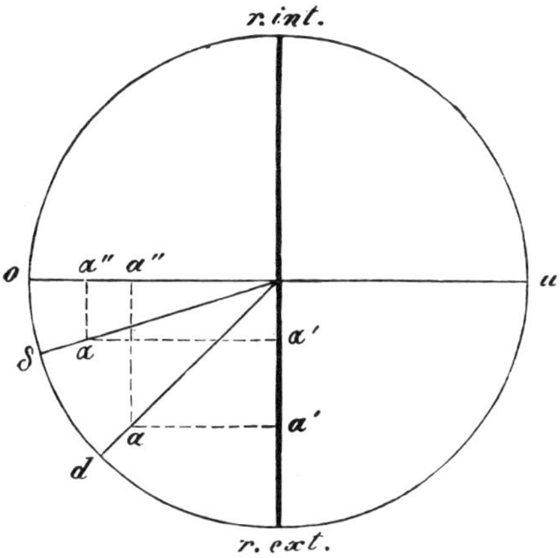

Fig. 28.

It is analogous with the moments of rotation which are necessary to elicit a diagonal movement from the primary position. Figure 28 is a vertical section of the left eye in the primary position coinciding with the primary axis plane. The radius labeled *r. int.* is the half axis of the medial rectus and the opposite radius is that of the lateral rectus. Given that the eye should begin a rotation about a half axis *md,* i.e., upward and to the left, the necessary moment of rotation (which we will label *ma*) can be thought of only as a resultant of two moments of rotation in the drawing, that is, in the primary axis plane. It is possible to elicit these two moments of rotation only on the one side by the lateral rectus and on the other side by the combined action of the two raisers, that is, that of the superior rectus and of the inferior oblique. Specifically, the movement elicited by the combined actions of the latter muscles must fall in the primary axis plane. This is possible only because it comes to lie in the half axis *mo*. Therefore, when the moment of rotation *ma″* results from the common tension of the two raisers, and the moment of rotation of the lateral rectus equals *ma′*, then the desired moment of rotation *ma* will finally result. Analogously, the moment of rotation *ma* would result from the two moments of rotation *ma′* and *ma″*. etc.

The combined tension of the lateral rectus, superior rectus, and inferior oblique is therefore necessary to begin a movement of the eye from the primary position upward and outward, no matter about which half axis of the relevant quadrant of the axis plane the rotation should occur. Further, the antagonistic relationship of the two pulling forces of the superior rectus on one side and the inferior oblique on the other must always be exactly the same, because the moment resulting from these two pulling forces must always fall in the axis plane itself; as figure 27 has shown, this is possible only with a single relationship of those pulling forces. The same now applies for the pulling forces of the two raisers when the movement is directed upward and inward; analogously it follows for the pulling forces of the two lowerers, the inferior rectus and the superior oblique.

We come then to the important result *that the antagonistic relationship of the pulling forces of the two lowerers must always be the same when with their participation the eye is to begin a rotation away from the primary position.* In other words, the two muscles must always be innervated with the same relationship, and a special determination of the innervation power for each single muscle according to the direction of the movement is not necessary. I had made the statement above that the superior rectus and the inferior oblique behave like a single muscle with respect to the innervating will, and that the same applies for the inferior rectus and the superior oblique. The above gives a proof for the correctness of that statement, though only for those movements which begin from the primary position. But this is not intended to decide rigorously that the two raisers or the two lowerers must also be equally strongly innervated, though this is likely in view of the very different sections of the two muscles; it should only be said that the way in which the two muscles are brought into play together is always the same, no matter which movement they participate in.

We have now determined the muscles involved in a rotation about a given half axis, as one would when the rotational force encountered either no resistances at all or only diametrically opposed ones. If we examine these resistances more exactly, we find that inward rotation opposes principally the lateral rectus, i.e., the pure antagonist of the now-innervated medial rectus. With horizontal rotation outward only the medial rectus significantly opposes the active lateral rectus. With vertical rotation upward or downward we find first the inferior rectus and superior oblique, and second the superior rectus and inferior oblique as the muscles which offer the significant resistances. Again, these are the muscles which antagonize the active ones. Finally, with oblique movements the three resisting muscles are always the antagonists of the three active ones. The moment of rotation resulting from the resistances of the stretched muscles may always be understood as rotational force approximately opposed to the active muscles, which therefore indeed inhibits the rotational force but cannot deviate it from its path.

But when the line of sight is away from the primary position, the two muscles which were exact antagonists in that position cease to remain so; in spite of this, their deviation from antagonism remains very small. If the muscles were elastic and anchored only at both end points, but were otherwise fully free threads, these deviations from Listing's Law could be exactly calculated. But because much more complicated relationships obtain in these muscles, because they lie on the eyeball with very wide tendons and can neither move freely along it nor move fully unhindered in the eye socket it is impossible to calculate the half axes of the rotational forces of the single muscles for secondary positions, i.e., the secondary half axes of the muscles. Nonetheless, meaningful conclusions can be drawn from the arrangement of muscles even in secondary positions.

Listing's Law, as we have seen, makes the cyclorotation during eye movements as small as possible. *Correspondingly, the momentary axes about which the eye is rotated never deviate significantly from the position at right angles to the line of sight, i.e., from the primary axis plane.* Consideration of the method of insertion of the eye muscles on the bulb teaches us further *that the half axes of rotational force of the single muscle, even at varying positions of the eye, do not deviate from their primary position.* From this it follows that to rotate the eye from a secondary position in one of the directions in which we have just moved the eye away from the primary position the muscles must be brought into action in an analogous way for the same direction: to move vertically upward, for instance, the pulling forces of the raisers must again stand in approximately the same antagonistic relationships. Of course it cannot be proved in this way that this analogy must be entirely strict; but it is clear that it must be approximately true. This is in agreement with our assumption that even at secondary positions both the two raisers and the lowerers are always innervated with the same relationships, just as a single muscle, and that in addition the innervation is the same with equal direction of movement, whether the movement occurs from the primary position or from a secondary position.

We now observe even more precisely the positions of the raisers and lowerers at various secondary positions; we find that the line of sight is located more inward as it approaches the plane which one can think of as lying through the two obliques, while it is more distant from the plane in which the superior and inferior rectus nearly lie. Conversely, the opposite is the case when the line of sight is more outward. The action of each of the four muscles considered here can be thought of as divided into one component which raises or lowers the line of sight and another which rolls the eye about the line of sight. The more the line of sight approaches the plane of the two oblique muscles, the more the raising or lowering action of an oblique increases; the opposite is the case with the other two muscles, the superior and inferior recti, whose raising or lowering action would decrease. All muscles would have the opposite behavior if the line of sight turns outward. From this it follows, as Wundt (29) has already shown, that the common action of the superior rectus and the inferior oblique results in a raising which always remains approximately the same independent of whether the eye is in the primary position or is directed inward or outward, because when in a secondary position inward or outward the component of the pulling force of one muscle for raising the eyes becomes smaller as the corresponding component of the other muscle grows, and vice versa. The analog must also apply to the two lowerers.

This yields the interesting result *that the two raising muscles always raise the eye approximately equally high with equal strength of innervation, independent of whether it moves from the primary position or from a position directed horizontally inward or outward.* Further, consider the case when the eye is raised a given amount vertically from the primary position, by the innervation of the two raisers. The line of sight will remain at about the same height when an additional innervation of the medial or lateral rectus elicits an inward or outward movement, as long as the innervation of the raisers continues with undiminished strength throughout the movement. The analogous argument applies to the lowerers. This stands in complete agreement with our assumption that one and the same innervation of the medial and lateral recti is adequate to rotate the eye horizontally inward or outward independent of whether the rotation occurs from the primary position or another position directed upward or downward, as long as the existing innervation of the raisers or lowerers is maintained.

When the line of sight is positioned horizontally inward, and thus lies nearer to the plane of the two obliques, not only will the pulling power components of the obliques increase during raising or lowering relative to the same innervation strength in the primary position, but the component rolling the eyes about the line of sight will decrease its pulling power. Conversely, the rolling component of the pulling power of the superior rectus or inferior rectus increases. If the two raisers now participate in the same relationships as they do for the purpose of raising the eye from the primary position, then the two components directed toward circular rotation will no longer be able to raise opposingly, but the rolling action of the superior rectus will dominate the opposing action of the inferior oblique. The result will be a rolling of the eyes about the line of sight, occurring together with a raising of the eyes such that the upper end of the previously vertical retinal meridian will rotate somewhat inward. The analog will occur for movement downward from an inward-directed secondary position, and for movement upward and downward from an outward-directed secondary position. *Thus in all cases the rolling of the eyes about the line of sight will be expected to be such that it truly occurs according to Listing's Law:* that is, another agreement with our assumption of an always equal innervation in spite of varying eye positions.

An important result of the arrangement is that raising or lowering of the eye is accomplished not by simple but by double muscles. If the eye had only a single raiser or lowerer, as it has only a single adductor and abductor, and if the first two ran backward parallel to the median plane and not downward and inward as do the true superior and inferior recti, then such raisers or lowerers would indeed be able to move the eye vertically away from the primary position, but could not do so from an inward or outward directed secondary position. Further, such a raiser of the previously horizontal and inwardly turned eye would rotate the eye not purely upward but diagonally upward and somewhat inward, and the lowerer would move it diagonally inward and downward. At the same time the amount of raising or lowering would become smaller and smaller with equally strong innervation of the raiser or lowerer, the further the eye had been deviated inward or outward at the beginning of the movement. By dividing the raisers and lowerers into two differentiated branches, one rectus and one oblique, a situation is reached where one and the same innervation of these muscles always leads to an approximately equally directed and equally large raising or lowering, whether the eye is to be moved inward or outward from the primary position or from a secondary position.

Thus if one asks how the six eye muscles must be brought into action so that the eye would move according to Listing's Law, one concludes that in every case they must be very nearly so innervated that they fulfill the laws of innervation given above. One can just as well approach the problem from the opposite direction and move to consideration of the eye musculature under the assumption of the correctness of that law of innervation. A purely mechanical consequence of this assumption is that the eye must move at least very nearly as it truly does, i.e., according to Listing's Law. Herein lies a very significant support for that assumption. Because of the complexity of the relationships, however, the desired proof cannot be reached with mathematical exactness either through the first or the second method. One must consider that even Listing's Law is not applicable with mathematical exactitude, but that even in the middle portions of fixation space with parallel eyes, for which our analysis has the strongest validity, Listing's Law does not apply exactly. Second, one must remember that the laws of innervation which I have given have numerous other significant supports, some of which have already been discussed while others remain to be discussed.

23. *On the Mechanical Relationships between the Bifixation and the Cyclorotary Position of the Eyes*

Previously the rectus muscles have been assigned the function of giving the eye the necessary direction while the obliques have been given the supplementary assignment of mediating the cyclorotation of the eye to that position which is necessary for the present direction of the line of sight in the interest of vision. A similar analysis has recently been espoused (although implicitly) by Helmholtz, who is of the opinion that the child when it learns to see voluntarily chooses the cyclorotary orientations of the retinas, and finally becomes accustomed to those which are the best according to a principle of orientation proposed by Helmholtz. The fact that the obliques significantly influence the orientation of the eye is the reason for the assumption, sometimes not clearly explicit, that the eye position derived for the purpose of focusing the line of sight receives a necessary correction by the special innervation of an oblique. Ordinarily an accustomed association between focusing and cyclorotating innervation must then be learned for every single fixation position. As already mentioned, Helmholtz also assumes an original independence of the motility of one eye from that of the other. From this it would follow that in addition to the learning of the correct focus and cyclorotation of each single eye, even the association between two innervations of *both* eyes which are simultaneously necessary in themselves, but are as varied as desired, would have to become habitual. Such hypotheses reveal themselves as superfluous if one considers the principles of operation of the single eye muscles more exactly.

Let us assume the case that the movements of the eye occur solely to give the line of sight the correct position with respect to objects, and that cyclorotary position does not matter. We then ask ourselves how the muscles must be controlled in order to serve the focus of the line of sight in the most efficient manner.

Given that the eye in primary position should be moved to a point lying horizontally to the left or to the right, only the lateral or medial rectus is available to mediate the movement. If the line of sight is moved sideways by one of these muscles from the primary position, the rotation can occur only about an axis nearly at right angles to the line of sight, because on one hand the half axes of the muscles just referred to are so positioned, and on the other hand the resistances which oppose the rotation (as just discussed) are diametrically opposite the rotation and thus can specify no significant deviation from the desired path. The result is therefore that the eye must follow Listing's Law during rotation inward or outward even if the subject does not control the orientation of the eye during this rotation. Rather, the orientation demanded by Listing's Law results entirely from itself if the desired movement of the line of sight is executed.

We shall now see how the movement of the line of sight considered to be the most efficient would raise and lower the eye. Only two muscles are in the disposition to raise the eye from the primary position. First, the inferior oblique alone could be innervated; thereby, in spite of a relatively large expenditure of muscle power, the line of sight would come forward only slightly because, apart from the resistances, the largest portion of the power would be wasted on the strong rolling of the eye. At the same time, the line of sight would go not exactly upward, but would deviate outward from the intended path. The subject would therefore have to innervate the medial rectus also in order to correct this deviation. With all of this he would be able to reach only such a small raising of the line of sight with such a relatively large effort that he would soon give up this method of raising, even more because the strong rolling of the eye about the line of sight would necessarily be opposed by a torsion on the optic nerve and other tensions.

Second, the superior rectus could be used for the purpose of raising the eye. One would fare better with the sole tension of this muscle, but even so one would not reach a pure raising of the eye. Rather, the line of sight would deviate inward and a large portion of the expended energy would be lost through the rolling of the eye determined by the superior oblique. In order to correct the inward deviation of the line of sight one would have to innervate the lateral rectus somewhat and thereby create a circumstance where the line of sight is raised perpendicularly even though the larger degrees of raising would demand a relatively large effort of the active muscles and would create other difficulties because of the strong rolling of the eye. Alternatively, if the subject combined the innervation of the superior rectus with that of the inferior oblique, he could accomplish a straight line raising of the line of sight and could raise the eye most efficiently without overloading either of the two muscles. What is therefore more natural than to assume that the subject would very soon come to use the muscle combinations just discussed for raising the eye if he did not already find them instinctively, that is, because of inborn innervation paths? But if the eye should be raised by the combined working of the superior rectus and the inferior oblique, it would thereby follow Listing's Law, for the best way of raising is always that by which the axis of rotation lies at right angles to the line of sight. In this way the entire moment of rotation is devoted to moving the line of sight, and nothing is lost to rolling of the eye about the line of sight. As we saw, the resistances which significantly oppose the raising of the eye using these muscles lie in the two antagonists of the latter and therefore cannot significantly deviate the rotation specified by the innervated muscles from its path. Here too the eye would behave according to Listing's Law even if the subject considers only the most efficient raising of fixation and does not consider orientation further.

Analyses entirely identical to those which we have given for raising the line of sight can be transferred to its lowering, and finally the analogous can be said for oblique movements of the line of sight away from the primary position. Everywhere we find that the subject when he wants to move the line of sight in the simplest and easiest way has no choice at all, but is strictly limited to entirely specified muscles and muscle combinations, for every attempt to execute a movement with other muscles must bring striking discomfort and difficulty with it.

Therefore, wherever the subject moves his line of sight from the primary position, even when he intends nothing more than the movement of the fixation point, he will nevertheless choose that innervation which the law of innervation given above demands, which then as a purely mechanical consequence always results in nearly that orientation which Listing's Law demands. Why then the assumption that we must especially study orientation and painstakingly seek a special orientation for every fixation, and then practice each of these hundreds of combinations? If we want to reach our next goal in the easiest and most comfortable possible way, that is to accomplish the transfer of fixation from one point to another, we can behave in no other way than we really do. Orientation according to Listing's Law, along with its numerous advantages for vision, is so to say a purely mechanical bonus which we receive without special efforts directed at it. The muscle system of the eyes is efficiently arranged from the beginning as is the organism in general; for were it not equipped for life and for the surmounting of difficulties which it finds everywhere then it could not indeed endure. The child who has learned to bend his arm at the elbow by innervation of the biceps involuntarily executes a useful supination of the hand for purely mechanical reasons. Nature also gives him the most efficient orientation of the eye if he correctly positions it on an object.

In my earlier publications on binocular vision I have indicated here and there that certain functions of the sense of sight find their basis in inborn arrangements. On this basis my opinion has been caricatured as though I let the child into the light of the world already completely educated as a visual virtuoso, and as though the images of external objects were shoved from the eyes onto the stage of consciousness fully complete in form and color like sets from the wings of a theatre. So I must fear that my above opinion that Listing's Law is already determined by the inborn mechanisms of the musculature will experience a similar misinterpretation, and it will be said that I treat the living muscle system of the eye with regard to the subject as though one set the dead mechanism of an automaton into movement through a few strings. In order to ameliorate this eventuality somewhat in advance, I will add the following.

The entire motor system of our body is apparently modifiable by experience in large degree, as much in its nervous as in its muscular part. The urge to movement indeed finds many inborn paths available in which the current of innervation flows especially easily, and many functional associations of various movements lie already formed in the organism of the newborn. But the will of the learner attempts to revise even the innervation of the less easily exercised paths and to come upon new paths for them; it attempts to rationalize given associations more or less and to establish new connections between various movements. The motor system of the eyes is surely no exception to this, and nothing opposes the assumption that it is possible for us to somewhat influence even the orientation of our eyes in their movements and to further extend the individual function of the system, which is basically predetermined by the entire arrangement of the musculature. But this will have its narrow limitations, even for the newborn, and much more for adults for whom in this context the case of paresis of one or another muscle gives us a striking proof of the narrow limits of such corrections.

In some animals the half axes of the obliques fall in the line of sight itself. If this were the case in humans, these muscles could much more plausibly have an extensive influence on cyclorotation. But when the obliques engage the eyeball they also move the line of sight significantly with their contraction. Each change of orientation brought about by these muscles brings with it a change of the direction of the eye, which must be further compensated by innervation of the recti. At least for distance accommodation it is nonetheless possible to voluntarily increase or decrease the divergence of the vertical dividing lines by small increases in innervation of the superior or inferior obliques. We must only take into consideration that this change of innervation is not unique for each direction of fixation, but is the same for all directions. It would also cause a change in the primary position. We could further think that the increasing divergence of the vertical dividing lines with increasing convergence of the lines of sight is determined by an equal innervation of the two inferior obliques, which the subject has become accustomed to in the interest of clear vision, because as we have seen this offers a significant optical advantage. But here too we may not forget that the innervation of the obliques cannot be chosen specially for each single near position, but that it is associated with the innervation of the adductor group. It increases and decreases with the convergence angle and must remain equally strong with constant innervation of the medial recti, as the investigation of the position of the dividing lines in near vision given above would also indicate.

All this may be assumed without coming into conflict with the facts. But to go further and assert that the newborn must learn a special orientation for every single eye position would stand in contradiction with all results of the investigations given above, and those who would assume it must deny the validity of the laws of innervation given above.

The observation of the eye movements of the newborn is associated with the hypothesis that not only the given association between the muscles of the same name in both eyes but also the association between each individual rectus and oblique muscle of the same eye is perhaps already given in the newborn. At least it has struck me that the eyes of the newborn do not simultaneously happen to change their angle of convergence, when they are raised or lowered, as would have to be the case if the raising or lowering of the eyes were mediated by isolated innervation of the corresponding rectus or oblique muscles. Although I do not want to put any special weight on this, it should indeed be reported, at least to show that the eye movements of the newborn offer nothing which can in any way be used to support the hypotheses which deny the inborn association of the eye muscles. Rather, everything speaks for these associations but nothing speaks against it.

Commentary on Part Three

In Chapter 20, *Background about the eye muscles,* Hering lays the groundwork for the discussion of mechanical aspects of eye movements. As indicated above in Part II, this Part III deals with the derivation of the law of innervation from the point of view of the mechanics of the eye muscles.

Hering first reviews the anatomical literature not only to discuss the location of the insertions of the eye muscles but also to emphasize that the eye muscles are not elastic threads but have broad insertions; they have the crucial effect of making the actions of the muscles insensitive to the position of the eyeball. The kinematic directions of the forces are analyzed starting with the consideration of each muscle separately, and developing a half-axis of rotation that would be produced if only a particular single muscle were activated. The resistive forces of the other five muscles and the passive elements of the eyeball are then accounted for. When the eye is stationary, the sum of the forces must be zero; Hering approaches several arguments in this kinematic chapter from the point of view of incremental analysis about stationary equilibria.

Hering (and indeed Helmholtz, his contemporary) were not on facile terms with dynamic effects. Their instrumentation and observational capabilities limited their intellectual attempts to come to grips with dynamical problems. There is some indication that Hering thought that tonic forces could be generated without active innervation, for he uses elastic tension sometimes as synonymous with dynamical force. There is an obvious lack of consideration of Descartes' Law of Reciprocal Innervation, although Charles Bell had already done his famous experiments. At that time Sherington was still thirty years away from his neurophysiological experimental confirmation. However, as we will see below, Hering does realize that antagonistic opposing forces occur in the same plane as the agonist (Chapter 22).

In Chapter 21, *On the single actions of the eye muscles,* Hering continues his discussion of the planes of action of the muscles and their half axes of rotation combined with consideration of the opposing resistance. He clearly states that single actions can never occur, since cyclorotation would be the inevitable result. Carefully exploiting his medical background, he points out that single paresis is an appropriate counter-example to this physiological argument since in these cases cyclorotation does occur.

Here we have another beautiful argument for innate laws of innervation as opposed to learning by experience; the subject with the paretic muscle never does compensate by learning to use his other five muscles so as to obtain the necessary three-degrees-of-freedom control of ocular rotation.

Hering points out that single action never occurs for the vertical muscles; they must be treated as a group. Again, reciprocal innervation is not considered in the action of the horizontal muscles. Finally, the independence of the horizontal and vertical muscular mechanisms is indicated; modern experimental evidence by T. Bahill and L. Stark has confirmed this with dynamical studies that prove Hering's point.

In Chapter 22, *On mechanical proofs for the innervation law given in Chapter 10,* Hering further develops his arguments in solid fashion. He states that in primary position since the agonist and antagonist forces are equal consequent to the requirement that the sum of forces must be zero, if one should cut all muscles, nothing would happen instantaneously. Next, a free choice of muscles does not exist; only one innervation is possible for each direction of gaze. With six muscles in three pairs acting in three planes we therefore have only three degrees of freedom. It is only possible to have minor forces in addition to these primary ones. Hering discusses the need for two vertical muscles for upward movements and for oblique or diagonal movements. Again, he makes the point that the four vertical muscles act as a single motor. He then extends his consideration to movements not starting in the primary position. Here he states that although deviations such as cyclorotations certainly are possible, they are minimized since the muscles are not threads but have broad insertions. For example, vertical combinations appear to be fixed and independent of horizontal gaze position; he refers to his own observations in this connection. Further, horizontal movements are independent of vertical gaze position.

Hering now gets into an argument which leads him into error because of his lack of consideration of Descartes' Law of Reciprocal Innervation. He discusses the problem of vertical elevation when horizontal gaze is directed inward, that is, in the adducted eye. In these circumstances, the IO will produce elevation but no excyclorotation, the SR will only elevate a little but will produce a considerable amount of incyclorotation and therefore some incyclorotation will occur. If we consider Descartes' Law of Reciprocal Innervation, we see that the IR and SO will be inhibited so that the excyclorotation of the IR will decrease (incyclorotation of the SO will be eliminated); thus any net cyclorotation would be minimized by reciprocal innervation. Clearly in more extreme positions, Listing's Law will be violated and only Donders' Law obeyed.

In this discussion, Hering appears to confuse true cyclorotation both with the false torsion that obtains concurrently with any diagonal movement and with the value of C_H, the cyclorotary term in Helmholtz' coordinate system for that triple coordinate set of values for which $C_L = 0$. Here C_L is cyclorotation in Listing's coordinate system and is equivalent to true cyclorotation.

Hering appreciates that the four vertical muscles act in a more elegant and effective fashion than if there were only two vertical rotators. This is analogous to the concept of the broad tendon acting to extend and spread muscular forces to reduce any effect of initial conditions of eyeball position. Thus since only second-order effects will obtain we need only a simple innervation law to obey Listing's Law.

In Chapter 23, *On the mechanical relationships between the bifixation and the cyclorotary position of the eyes,* Hering starts by mentioning the old theory that the oblique muscles were responsible for cyclorotations and that it was necessary for each human to learn the appropriate cyclorotations for each direction of gaze. He opposes these old theories and suggests a simple argument, considering first only how to control the direction of gaze. We need only that fixed pattern of innervation for which minimum force changes are required and for which *no* cyclorotation occurs. This is certainly true for horizontal and vertical movements since axes of rotation are orthogonal to the line of sight and therefore no cyclorotation can occur. It is equivalent to the geometrical statement of Listing's Law. We can now extend this to any oblique direction of rotation: the axes of rotation stay in Listing's plane and no cyclorotations occur. Thus, we don't in fact have to learn any cyclorotation.

Hering mentions that biceps contraction both flexes the elbow and produces hand supination, a useful kinematic combination. Here he inserts his famous plea against being caricatured (see introduction). He agrees that some learning with experience can take place but only within narrow limits. Again, he takes the case of the paretic muscle to demonstrate how difficult, indeed, it is to change coordination by learning. Two further observations are that the oblique muscles do not have axes of rotation that fall on the line of sight, as in some lower animals such as fish; and finally that he has not observed vergence in response to vertical movements of newborns. We may interpret this latter statement as a suggestion that Hering might well have wanted to integrate the laws of innervation of the single eye with the law of innervation for binocular movements.

Part IV. On the Accommodation of the Double Eye

24. *On the Equal Innervation of Both Eyes*

The intraocular muscles, which mediate accommodation for the present distance of the observed object and the amount of light coming into the eye, have the same equality of innervation of both eyes which is found in the extraocular muscles. In the same way, be it through reflex or through innervation released by the will, these muscles act equally strongly in both eyes at the same time. In these focusing movements we find an even closer association of both eyes than we have come to know for the positioning movements.

The eyes of a normal-sighted person are generally always accommodated for that point on which the lines of sight are focused. One accommodation suffices for *both* eyes. The fixated point usually is almost equally distant from both eyes, and further one and the same state of refraction permits (as is known) a certain tolerance within which it can move further or nearer without yielding noticeable blur (Czermak's accommodation line). Only when the fixated point is very near and to one side does this no longer apply. Given that the lines of sight have the position illustrated in Figure 29, the fixated object O will lie considerably nearer to the right eye than to the left. The right eye will therefore need a stronger accommodation than the left. Nevertheless, such an inequality of accommodation does not occur because we are not able to accommodate one eye more strongly than the other; rather, every accommodative innervation always applies to both eyes equally.

Thus, if I fixate a pin in the position just described (Figure 29) and by slight squinting split its image into two images lying very close to one another, only one image, that of the right eye, appears sharp to me, while that of the left appears in blur circles. Conversely, the image of the left eye appears sharp if the object is to the left and therefore lies nearer to the left eye. Because this experiment succeeded for me on both sides, it follows that its result cannot be due to my left eye being somewhat more shortsighted than the right. One who is myopic and can strongly converge will receive an especially striking result, because one can obtain a larger difference of object distance from both eyes the nearer one brings the object to the eye.

In the eye position described, bring two identical pins b and b' to the distance where one is exactly as far from the left eye as the other is from the right (as the figure shows). Then split the originally single fused image of the two pins into two images again by a small change of the convergence angle. Both pins will appear without blur, which shows that both eyes are equally strongly accommodated. One who does not have very good control of his eyes would do well in these experiments to divide the single image with a weak prism, which he holds with the base upward or downward in front of the eye. Then one must only substitute other objects for the fine pins, for instance fine holes stuck into opaque paper, because the superimposed double images of the pins would partly cover one another.

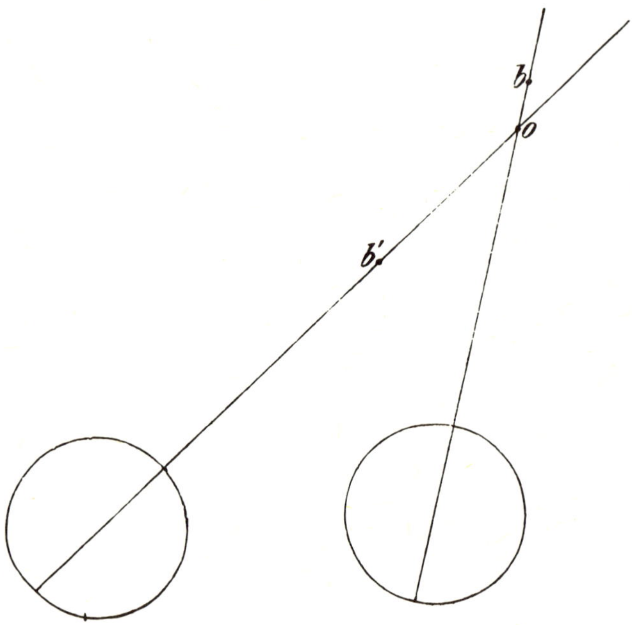

Fig. 29.

If one sees with only one eye while the other is covered, and accommodates the seeing eye for nearness, then the covered one also accommodates in entirely the same way, as the practiced observer can immediately recognize if he suddenly removes the cover from the other eye.

It is known that the pupil becomes smaller during accommodation for nearness. This decrease too, as well as the enlargement, always occurs simultaneously and equally strongly in both eyes. If one sticks a fine hole in a strong sheet of paper and brings it very near to the eye, one sees the hole, as is known, as a small lighted disc whose size (*ceteris paribus*) depends on the size of the pupil and increases and decreases with it. If one fixes the head and brings a small fixed screen with a small hole very close to each eye, and so arranges the lines of sight that each goes through a hole in the screen on the corresponding side, then the images from the two holes will fuse into a single one. If one now sticks a hole in one screen just above the first hole, and just below in the other, one receives three images with binocular fusion of the first two holes, as three small light discs lying over one another. The middle one is seen binocularly while the upper and lower ones are each seen from only one eye. One can now easily so arrange it that the upper and the lower discs appear exactly equal in size. If one now changes accommodation without disturbing the lines of sight, one sees the upper and the lower disc simultaneously and equally strongly becoming larger or smaller. Of course, it is necessary to have the proper practice in changing accommodation adequately with stationary eye position. According to the position which one gives to the two small screens, one can do this experiment at any desired eye position and be convinced that under all circumstances both pupils become larger or smaller at the same time and to the same degree.

The involuntary movements of the iris by which the eye adapts to the present light level behave like the voluntary movements of the iris in accommodation. Whether the light stimulus meets only one or both retinas, the iris reflex is always exercised in the same way in both eyes; both pupils become larger or smaller at the same time and in the same amount. One can show this with an experiment entirely analogous to the previous one. The two screens are arranged such that they darken the eye as much as possible, and the four fine holes are aligned exactly as before. In one screen one makes a larger window outward from the two fine holes, which can be closed or opened to any desired degree with a cover. If one now directs the gaze at the holes in the screen in the manner described above and suddenly opens the window of the one screen so that an adequate amount of light falls on the peripheral retina of the corresponding eye, then one sees a simultaneous and equal decrease in the size of the upper and lower of the three lighted discs: a proof that the light stimulus falling on the retina elicited a reflex innervation of both irises which was equally strong and simultaneous on the two sides.

It is of great interest that with this involuntary innervation the eye behaves quite similarly to the voluntary situation, namely as two parts of a whole directed by a single innervation.

Donders had already shown that both pupils constrict simultaneously when one stimulates one eye with light, in contrast to Listing, according to whom the consensual contraction in the unstimulated eye began somewhat later than that in the directly stimulated one. "If one places a convex lens in front of the eye and looks at a distant point of light, one sees an illuminated disc whose form and size depend on the form and size of the pupil. If one now sets a convex lens in front of each eye, one somewhat higher than the other, one sees both pupils above one another and can comfortably compare them." (6)

25. *On the Relationship between Accommodation and Convergence*

Because the eyes of a person with normal vision are always accommodated for the present distance of the point of sight, it was assumed earlier, especially on the authority of Johannes Müller, that there was a fixed relationship between accommodation and convergence of the lines of sight. Later E.H. Weber (28), Volkmann (27), Donders (4), and others showed that one can change accommodation somewhat with constant convergence, and recently Helmholtz (14) has described the relationship between the two as only a habit.

In adults, the innervation of the accommodation muscles doubtless has a forced association to the innervation of the adductor group of the double eye. Therefore, only when the two medial recti are simultaneously innervated to bring the point of sight closer does innervation for accommodating the eyes occur. Innervation of the sideward turners is in no way linked to the change of accommodation of the eye whose medial rectus is thereby innervated. If the eyes converge for instance on a nearby point to the right, the left medial rectus is shortened and the right one is indeed lengthened; at the same time, both eyes are accommodated for nearness, and as was indicated in chapter 2, both adductors of the double eye are innervated even if both are not shortened. Only in the light of the law of always equal innervation of the double eye is it justified to speak of a synergy between the medial recti and the accommodation muscles. The previous understanding of this relationship was adequate as long as the eyes converged symmetrically, but not when the fixation point lay unsymmetrically to the left or to the right. Here also it is true that both eyes are always equally strongly accommodated even when, as shown above, this does not correspond to the position of the object. The double eye is organized as a whole for near vision with both medial recti, both ciliary muscles, and both irises simultaneously and equally strongly innervated. In no way is each eye alone adjusted to the position of the object. *There exists, therefore, no relationship between the contraction of the medial rectus of one eye and its accommodation, but there is a relationship between the innervation of the adductor group and the innervation of the accommodation muscle of the double eye.*

Like most associations of movement, the one referred to here indeed applies within specific boundaries but is never completely dissociable. The range within which accommodation can be varied with constant convergnece of the lines of sight, that is the relative accommodation distance (Donders), shows large individual differences. The unpracticed subject is able to free his accommodation somewhat from convergence only with the help of artificial procedures which will be discussed immediately below. This is possible for the practiced, as E.H. Weber has shown even without any apparatus. When he fixated a far point he could accommodate the eye for greater nearness and could suppress the accompanying strong urge for increasing of convergence, eliminate the accompanying crossed double images, and also see the fixated point in blur circles. In the same way, he could call forth blur during fixation of a near point by ceasing accommodation.

The possibility to free the association between direction and focus somewhat is of the greatest importance when in the course of life either the state of refraction or the form of the eyeball changes, when the ability to accommodate weakens, or when the outer movement apparatus of the eye suffers small disturbances.

Suppose that a normally sighted person begins to become myopic: he will now expend a smaller innervation for the purpose of proper accommodation of the eye during convergence of the lines of sight than earlier, and he would not be able to see clearly any more if the dissociation of his previously functional association of focus and direction innervation were not possible to some degree. Someone who is hypermetropic would behave in an analogous way. Expanded further, with otherwise unchanged relationships the accommodation apparatus for some reason or another responds with a smaller degree of accommodation for the same strength of innervation as earlier. The subject then would need to apply a stronger innervation than before in order to reach the accommodation corresponding to the convergence of the lines of sight. Finally, if one or both adductors or abductors of the double eye for some reason no longer react with the same energy as earlier for the same innervation, then the subject will find necessary a stronger innervation of these muscles in order to reach a given eye position. But the innervation for focusing would not be able to increase or decrease correspondingly, because it would not then correspond to the eye position.

The stronger the demands which are made through these anomalies for releasing the relationship of the two relevant innervations, and the less time the patient is given to become accustomed to them, the more strenuous clear vision will become. The situation can develop which is known under the name of asthenopy. If the demands exceed the always very limited possibility of modification the patient will be forced to give up either clear vision or binocular vision; he must either see poorly or squint.

26. *On the Artificial Dissociation of the Relationship between Accommodation and Convergence*

If someone holds a weak prism before the eye with its vertical base outward he sees crossed double images at first, but they are soon single again because he eliminates the double images by an increase in the convergence of the eyes. If he uses a strong prism for the same experiment, when he is not practiced in the observation of peripheral double images, he does not see double but does see various things unclearly through one another. He sees a different part of visual space with each eye and is not able to reestablish clear vision unless he finds the necessary eye position by chance. The observer who is practiced in such experiments indeed immediately notices the corresponding double image for each image, if it is at all recognizable, and easily reestablishes single vision by strong convergence. In this way I myself have overcome every prism which does not demand a stronger inward turning of the eye than the anchoring of the eyeball permits.

When the unpracticed person holds a weak prism with the vertical base inward and observes a very distant object, he sees double but cannot untie the double images at all or can do so only with great difficulty. He cannot bring forth the divergence of the lines of sight which is necessary for single vision but is quite unaccustomed to him. The nearer the observed object lies, the stronger the prism which he can overcome. But if one holds a strong prism in front of one eye in the way described, then he again sees various parts of visual space unclearly through one another. The practiced observer, however, does not see double through a prism so arranged even if it is strong, and succeeds in overcoming every prism which demands only a reduction of convergence; indeed, it is known that after some practice even prisms which demand a measureable divergence of the lines of sight can be mastered.

If I look into the far distance, hold a prism base outward in front of one eye and then let the double images go together slowly so to say by themselves, I see, if the angle of the prism exceeds a certain size, that the observed object in the first moment is always less clear than before. Indeed, the effect is stronger the faster the double images move together, but is strongest if I fuse them very quickly voluntarily so that I cannot observe anything about the two images during the movement. This unclearness is soon lost again inasmuch as it is not determined purely physically by the prism *to the degree that the prism does not exceed a certain strength, in which case the unclarity is lasting.* This no longer compensatable unclarity is not simply a result of the disturbed retinal images from the astigmatic action of the prism, but is a result of inappropriate accommodation for nearness. I conclude this without doubt because if I quickly cover the equipped eye so that the object is now seen only with the unequipped eye and still appears unclear, it very soon becomes sharper and sharper while making an apparent movement inward. Further, after quick covering of the unequipped eye, the object seen through the prism similarly becomes sharper while experiencing an apparent inward movement until finally only a small unclarity remains which is caused by the achromatic and astigmatic action of the prism. Both eyes have therefore accommodated for nearness as a result of the onesided squint, and the compulsion for this accommodation is so great that I cannot overcome it in spite of all practice.

Everything behaves quite analogously when I fixate a very close object and then hold a prism with the base inward in front of one eye. The force for minimizing accommodation characterizes itself in entirely the same way, but is finally overcome within specific boundaries. On the other hand, if the prism is even stronger a constant accommodation for too great a distance occurs in spite of all efforts, and both eyes are permanently accommodated for a larger distance than is expressed by the position of the fixated object.

The prism therefore induces an accommodation in both eyes which corresponds to the increase or decrease of the convergence which it determines. A false accommodation can indeed be compensated to a certain degree by a voluntary opposite impulse, though this cannot be exceeded.

Accompanying the accommodation changes in these experiments is a corresponding change in pupil diameter, also in both eyes, as one can be convinced by a second person. But this observation is easy to make only on those who have some practice in physiological-optical experiments, for novices often throw their eyes back and forth so unsteadily in the urge for clear vision that one cannot follow the changes of the pupil while they occur, but must constitute them through two comparative measurements, which is more complicated.

The simultaneous change of accommodation and pupil size in *both* eyes stands in agreement with the simultaneous innervation of *both* medial or lateral recti, which can be assumed in these experiments as well as in earlier experiences. *The deviation of one eye does not occur because its medial or lateral rectus is innervated on one side;* rather, the sequence is quite analogous to that which was given in Chapter 4, which was concerned with alternate binocular fixation of two points on the line of sight of one eye with unchanged position at various distances.

If, instead of one prism, one puts a prism of half as large an angle in front of each eye, first with the base upward or downward, and then slowly rotates both prisms in opposite directions until both bases lie vertically outward or inward, then it is easier for the unpracticed person to succeed in seeing singly through the prims than if he immediately places both prisms with the bases vertical or uses only one prism of doubled strength with a vertical base. In the first case the double images are pulled only slightly away from one another and therefore they always excite a new stimulus for single vision. But one must carefully rotate both prisms with equal speed; otherwise double images superimposed on one another will appear which the unpracticed can hardly unify at all.

In all of these experiments the convergence of the lines of sight does not correspond to the distance of the observed object, given that it is seen singly with both eyes. On the contrary, the line of sight of the equipped eye goes outward past the observed object if the base of the prism lies inward, and inward when the prism is reversed. It is now a question of how accommodation behaves under these conditions and whether it changes parallel to the increase or decrease in convergence.

Generally, as I will show, this is definitely the case even though the natural and involuntary urge to the accustomed accommodation can be overcome within certain limits, as Donders has already indicated. I have made my accommodation range relatively quite independent of the convergence of the lines of sight by many exercises according to various methods, but I must assert with respect to these opposing opinions that my prism-induced squint always gives a natural inducement for a change of accommodation, which cannot be overcome when it exceeds a certain amount.

When we observe a distant point with both eyes and then bring a prism with its vertical base outward in front of the left eye, a compulsion or a voluntary intention to converge arises because of the crossed double images. The corresponding innervation occurs simultaneously in both eyes, as both begin to move inward. But because the right eye is now the only fixation one, in that only it still sees the object directly, and because the deviation of this eye inward due to the above innervation moves the image of the observed object from the middle of the retina inward, there follows immediately a second innervation to turn the double eye in order to prevent the deviation of the fixating eye to the left and to hold the object in direct vision. These two innervations now exist simultaneously with periodic dominance of one over the other until the left eye is adequately turned inward and binocular single vision is again achieved. The medial rectus of the left eye is thus innervated with double strength, first because of the innervation of the adductor group directed toward convergence and second because of the innervation directed to sideward turning of the double eye. The right eye similarly stands under this doubled innervation; it is pulled inward by one and outward by the other, and the opposition of both influences as well as the periodic dominance of one over the other betrays itself, especially in the unpracticed, by a back and forth oscillation of the unequipped eye.

If the other innervation were not there, the innervation for rightward turning would itself rotate both eyes through half of that angle through which the left eye actually rotates to the right. Corresponding to that innervation for turning binocular fixation to the right there now occurs an additional apparent movement of the fixated object, which will be thoroughly discussed later.

It is known that another aid in making accommodation somewhat independent of convergence is eyeglasses. The person with normal vision should attempt to see clearly into the distance through very weak concave glasses, first only with effort and after a while more easily; it is similar for nearness with very weak convex glasses. But difficulties arise as soon as the glasses are too strong, and finally the strong urge for proper accommodation induces a deviation of one eye inward if concave glasses are used and outward if convex glasses are used, because the focusing innervation is involuntarily associated with innervation of the outer eye muscles. One eye then deviates enough that the convergence angle of the lines of sight corresponds to the degree of accommodation necessary for clear vision. One then fixates the object, however, with only one eye and is somewhat bothered by the competition of the visual fields, though he nevertheless sees better than before.

Finally, a convergence not corresponding to accommodation can be obtained without prism or lenses with the help of stereoscopic images. Depending on the distance from the eye and the distance at which one places the two separated halves of a stereoscopic double image and fuses them (with crossed or uncrossed lines of sight), one can induce a disharmony between the eye position and the distance of the images from the eyes. A convergence not corresponding to accommodation is then necessary in order to see clearly. In this way one can change accommodation with constant convergence just as well as change convergence with constant accommodation, while convincing oneself here also that this is possible only within very narrow limits.

Until now in the determination of relative accommodation range (Donders (5) and MacGillavry (20)), a significant fact has been overlooked (as has already been touched upon above). With lowering of the fixation plane the eyes involuntarily converge. Because this urge for convergence is purely mechanically based and is not accomplished by innervation of the medial recti, it is not accompanied by a corresponding increase in accommodation tension. Thus it happens that in myopes, for instance with me, that the binocular far point is further away with a fixation plane lowered relative to the heaa than with a horizontal or even with a raised fixation plane. For with a lowered fixation plane the medial recti achieve the same convergence of the lines of sight with a smaller innervation than with a raised plane, and the lateral recti must be correspondingly innervated. The innervation of the adductor group associated with innervation of the accommodation muscles is therefore less or disappears entirely. Because of this, *the position and range of binocular accommodation depth varies to the degree that it is determined by one or another head position with one or another position of the fixation plane.*

27. *On the Origin of the Relationship of Accommodation and Convergence*

I come to a question which is of highest importance, especially for pathology, aside from its physiological interest. The issue is whether the association between the innervations of the medial muscles and certain lateral muscles of the double eye are inborn or are established by long habit. The importance of the differentiation, as one will remember, throws light on the fact that myopia and hypermetropia are already apparent in the first years of childhood. The hypermetropic child must accommodate even with parallel lines of sight in order to see clearly, and with converging lines of sight he must accommodate much more strongly than is necessary for emmetropes, while the myopic child conversely need not let accommodation grow when converging with near vision in the same way as the normal person. If the association in question were not inborn, neither hypermetropes nor myopes would find difficulty in vision for objects of sight within their monocular accommodation range. Even with relatively small convergence of the lines of sight, the hypermetrope could call forth the higher degrees of accommodation tension without difficulty, while the myope in spite of strong convergence of the lines of sight would not be burdened by using his accommodation muscles very little or not at all.

The phenomena would be quite different if the association in question were inborn. The myopes as well as the hypermetropes would have to struggle against it, and even if the young organism because of its great flexibility succeeded in dissociating the association to a certain degree, it would be possible only slowly and with difficulty; during this time hypermetropes would necessarily have a great tendency toward inward squint and myopes toward outward squint. In order to see clearly the hypermetropes would always have to accommodate strongly with the innervation necessary for this, the innervation of the adductor group. A tendency to converge would set in and the temptation would arise to give up binocular vision in order to see the observed object clearly at least with one eye. The other eye would therefore deviate, and all the sooner if one of those fortunate moments were added as Donders has discussed them. The myope, on the other hand, because he can obtain sharp images only from near objects, would have to converge strongly; the innervation of the medial recti would be irrevocably linked with that of the accommodation muscles, his eye would thereby become even more shortsighted, and if the struggle against this compulsion burdened him too much he would give up the innervation of the medial recti. He would at least be able to see sharply with the fixating eye, though one eye would then indeed squint outward. He would grasp this solution even earlier if other further advantageous circumstances occur in addition, such as the mechanical difficulty of convergence or less sharp vision in one eye.

Donders has made us aware how frequently *strabismus internus* occurs in hypermetropes and *strabismus externus* in myopes. He has sought to explain the fact that the above refraction anomalies so often lead to squinting, especially when they are inborn, partly because of the relationship between accommodation and convergence of the lines of sight. This explanation would be unnecessary as I see it if this relationship were not inborn. But it would be just as unnecessary if an inborn compulsion for always equal innervation of both eyes did not occur. For how would it be conceivable for instance to assume, along with accommodation for nearness, a simultaneous compulsion for increasing the convergence of the lines of sight, if the child were free to move one eye outward or inward independently from the other? Thus if Donders' explanation is correct, it is also a convincing proof not only that the law of the always equal innervation of both eyes given above is correct, but also that this law is grounded in inborn mechanisms.

Most opthalmologists now agree that Donders correctly grasped the association in question as a significant cause of squinting with refraction errors. Even the single fact that the beginning strabismus internus of hypermetropic children can be cured by appropriate convex glasses is an adequate proof. Other facts are indeed available to support the assumption of an inborn relationship between the focusing innervation and the innervation of the adductors.

Donders and MacGillavry have determined the binocular accommodation range of various myopes and hypermetropes. It is quite generally true that the absolute near point of the hypermetropes is nearer to the eye than their binocular near point, that is, although *it would be necessary for clear vision, they never use their full accommodation capabilities with binocular vision.* They could do this only if they also gave the eyes a convergence that was too large in comparison to the position of the fixation point, as they in fact do in monocular vision. They are therefore not capable of fully dissociating the relationship between accommodation and convergence. To give an especially striking example, it is said that Donders (5, p. 202) described a relative hypermetropy in which the patient, a 17-year-old girl, *could never accommodate for the distance of the fixated object if she saw binocularly, although the near point of her two eyes singly was only ten inches from her face.* If she could make accommodation independent of convergence she would have been able to see everything sharply up to about one foot.

Conversely, it was found that the absolute far point of myopes was more distant from the eye than their binocular far point, that they therefore were more nearsighted with binocular vision than would have been the case had they been able to fully suppress the compulsion for accommodation in spite of convergence of the lines of sight. These are striking proofs of the permanence of the association. Because they are mostly concerned with congenital refraction errors, they also prove that this association is inborn and not acquired.

Helmholtz has not made note of this entire area of facts, for he makes the assertion that accommodation associates itself with convergence only through learning. His proof for this opinion is restricted to mention of the fact that the relationship of both abilities can be somewhat reduced artificially. I have already shown above that this proves nothing because it also applies to many other reflexes which are doubtless inborn.

28. *Pathology*

The facts that both eyes are always equally innervated, that an increase in accommodation occurs with innervation of the adductors and a decrease with innervation of the abductors, and that conversely every voluntary change of accommodation elicits a change in innervation of the lateral or medial recti, are of greatest importance for the theory of motility disturbances. In the previous paragraphs it has already been shown how this relationship between focusing and positioning innervation can lead to squint in myopia and hypermetropia. Here the meaning of that association will be briefly mentioned in cases of paralysis and paresis of single eye muscles, because the opthalmologists have not yet directed their attention to this point. Let us take the case of paresis of the left lateral rectus. If the paresis develops slowly and the affected muscle has not yet changed its elasticity significantly, then there will be a tendency to see uncrossed double images with distant vision in the left half of visual space. In order to bring these again into fusion the patient will innervate both lateral recti and initially will still see singly with increased effort. If he is also hypermetropic and must accommodate even with parallel lines of sight, the innervation of the lateral recti will be accompanied by a reduction of the state of refraction. He will therefore be troubled not only by the appearance of double images but also by blur which occurs as soon as he again gets rid of the double images. Therefore, because he will very soon no longer be able to obtain the accommodation necessary for sharp vision in addition to innervation of the lateral recti, he must give up either sharp vision or binocular vision.

But if the patient is myopic he can use innervation of the lateral recti to abolish the double images just as well as an emmetrope, if the paresis is still very weak, without seeing distant objects worse than before.

Now let us see how these relationships are arranged with near vision in the left half of visual space. If the patient is emmetropic he will at first find no significant disturbance with symmetrical near vision. But if he looks to the left and innervates the left turners for this purpose, his left lateral rectus will remain behind his right medial rectus in its action and therefore an unusually small innervation of the adductors will be adequate for focusing the lines of sight on the near point. This innervation, too weak in comparision to the eye position, will bring with it a corresponding deficit of accommodation tension, and the patient will have to make an effort to achieve an accommodation which exceeds the normal innervation state of the medial recti. To a certain degree this will be possible for him; he will behave as though a concave lens or a weak prism had been brought in front of one eye. But if the available innervation of the medial recti corresponding to the binocular accommodation range is exhausted, he will have to give up either sharp vision or binocular single vision.

If the patient is hypermetropic he will encounter this dismal alternative even sooner; conversely, if he is myopic a slight paresis of his lateral rectus will permit him to see objects clearly at a greater distance than before, and his binocular far point will extend out to the distance of the absolute far point.

The hypermetrope will therefore feel noticeable difficulties even with a beginning insufficiency of one lateral rectus, while the emmetrope suffers less and the myope is to a degree even better off than before. Weak convex glasses will significantly alleviate the difficulties of a normally sighted person and stronger ones will of course help the hypermetrope. An increase in the paresis will affect the condition of the hypermetrope most strongly, the emmetrope less, and the myope the least, and *the area of double vision will correspondingly be quite different even though the degree of paresis can be exactly the same in all three cases.*

The excursion ability of the affected eye will be more restricted the nearer the object is and the more strongly the patient must therefore accommodate. The largest restriction will therefore be shown by the hypermetrope. For when the eye is accommodated for nearness the lateral rectus encounters a larger resistance (in comparison with the simultaneously innervated medial rectus) than it would with a relaxed accommodation muscle; it will be able to rotate the eye correspondingly less. Therefore, with hypermetropes one can estimate the degree of deficit from this fact.

Conversely, if the medial rectus has paresis everything in general behaves oppositely; the hypermetrope is in a good position and notices his problem less while the myope is worst hit and the area of double vision is the largest for him.

It has previously been thought that with unsymmetrical near vision the medial rectus of one eye is either not innervated at all or is innervated more weakly than that of the other, and it has not been noticed that the eye is doubly innervated in this case. An unequal innervation of two associated sideward turners has been assumed in pathological cases as well. It is indeed conceivable that a dissociation of the central association of two such muscles is possible within certain boundaries; but I believe that I have brought forth adequate proof above that this effect cannot be very great.

Several hypotheses have been proposed to explain the so varied size of the area of diplopia in cases where one has no reason to assume a correspondingly varied degree of paresis; I will not judge their justification. It seems quite likely to me, however, that these hypotheses would not have been proposed if the relationships just discussed and the refraction condition of the eyes had been considered.

It is understood that what I have discussed here in a single example *mutatis mutandis* can find application whenever the balance between medial and lateral recti is disturbed, for some reason, as well as when such disturbances can be relieved by an operation or otherwise. The diagnosis and prognosis as well as the therapy of many motility disturbances will, in my opinion, reach a greater precision in the future if the refraction condition has a part in the judgement. The use of concave or convex glasses will thus appear beneficial in many cases of motility disturbance where they have not previously been prescribed.

In chapter 24, *On the equal innervation of both eyes for accommodation and pupillary movements,* Hering asserts that the intraocular muscles observe Hering's Law as fully as the extraocular muscles. Further, the same equality of innervation applies whether it drives a reflex movement or an 'innervation released by the will.'

Right and left eyes have equal accommodation states even though the two desired goals, the bifixation point and the accommodative distance, may not be equal, especially with near lateral gaze. Of importance here, as he points out, is a depth of focus tolerance in accommodation.

Hering illustrates this with four elegant experiments using the perception of different blur circles when unequal distances to a pin target make it impossible for the equally innervated accommodation mechanism of each eye to focus clearly the different target distances. Next, with two pins, he obtains two sharp images providing they are equi-distant from *each* eye. Then with a beautiful entoptic experiment, perceiving the binocular pupillary diameters, he shows how precisely the iris is also equally innervated. He thus favors Donders, who had previously shown that the consensual pupil always equals the direct pupil, over Listing, who suggested that the consensual pupil response had longer latency.

In chapter 25, *On the relationship betwen accommodation and convergence,* Hering attributes to Johannes Müller the discovery of the fixed accommodative convergence to accommodation (ACA) ratio and then mentions that Weber, Volkmann and Donders had showed that accommodation was somewhat changeable with fixed vergence. Helmholtz had asserted incorrectly that the ACA relationship is only a habit.

Hering's Law here states that vergence is linked simultaneously to accommodation by equal innervation. Both left medial rectus and right medial rectus are simultaneously related to accommodation. The innervation for version is not linked to accommodation so that when we consider asymmetrical vergence we must consider the consequences of that aspect of Hering's Law which asserts the independent summing action of version and vergence that allows any possible bifixation point to be achieved by the double eye. Thus on looking at a near point to the right, the RMR is relaxed and lengthened by the RLR and yet there is positive accommodation.

Left and right accommodation are strongly linked as are both pupils, so that they contract simultaneously and equally.

He quotes Donders on relative accommodation, stressing the large individual variations found, and Weber on how practice can increase relaxation of the fixed synkinetic ACA ratio. Hering points out that this minimal freeing of the ACA ratio becomes important with changes in the refractive state or with eye movement paresis.

The stronger and the quicker the sensory demands for anomalous ACA value the more strenuous the attempt for clear single vision becomes. This may yield asthenopia, or such resolution of the struggle as clear vision with squint, or single vision with blur.

In chapter 26, *On the artificial disassociation of the relationship between accommodation and convergence,* Hering discusses a set of experiments with prisms, and he is more often concerned with convergence accommodation than with accommodative vergence.

Through these prism adaptation experiments Hering shows that one can somewhat overcome the urge to accommodate. But he agrees with Donders that the natural inducement to accommodation, if large enough, cannot be overcome. He also discusses the crucial regions at the borders of the zone of single, clear binocular vision where blurring or diplopia may occur. He describes some insightful findings, such as his observation of the pupils changing concurrently with accommodation, still another aspect of Hering's Law. A further observation of Hering's is an 'oscillation' of the non-prismatic eye faced with conflicting cues in a prism-induced asymmetrical vergence, which of course calls forth both versional and vergence components in the response. This is perhaps the first observation of the saccade in asymmetrical vergence in the line-of-sight fixating eye. Hering discusses innervation of the medial rectus with double innervation strength and the lateral rectus with opposing innervation; this relates to the issue of whether cancellation occurs in the neural nuclei or mechanically on the globe.

Hering goes on to discuss the restricted regions within which accommodation and vergence can change in a non-corresponding way using glasses, prisms, or the stereoscope; his main observation here is the *small* discordant range.

In chapter 27, *On the origin of the relationship of accommodation with convergence,* Hering raises a most important question of the innate nature of the linking between the intraocular and extraocular muscles of the double eye. It is clear that when we consider myopia and hyperopia in children, a great deal of the consequent difficulty is due to the inborn nature of this association, which we may state as a further form of Hering's Law. The intense struggle to gain even a small dissociation is evidence for the innate and fixed nature of the ACA and CAC relationships.

The hyperope, using excessive accommodation, develops esotropia. He then gives up binocular vision, choosing to see clearly with one eye and allowing the other eye to deviate.

The myope develops exotropia. He then attempts strong convergence minimizing accommodation and becomes even more myopic. He then may give up innervation of one medial rectus (convergence) and get an outward squint (intermittent exotropia), but then see clearly with the fixating eye. He would seize this monocular situation if, in addition to the myopia, he had difficulty with convergence or had less sharp vision in one eye.

Hering attributes to Donders these associations between hyperopia and myopia and esotropia and exotropia as explained by the inborn ACA and CAC ratios. Hering states that children must have inborn equal innervation of both eyes, since the eyes cannot move independently and thus the corresponding innervation must also be inborn. Most ophthalmologists agree with Donders that the inborn association of the ACA ratio is a significant factor in squint with refractive errors.

Hering points to some further studies related to the monocular and binocular near and far points to show that the innate association of the extra- and intraocular muscles cannot be overcome even in pathological conditions. For example, with hyperopia the absolute monocular near point lies closer than the binocular near point (Donders and MacGillavry). Thus accommodation cannot be used to its full extent because overconvergence would ensue. Similarly, in the myope the absolute accommodative far point lies further than the binocular accommodative far point since in the latter case to relax accommodation would cause divergence and diplopia.

These are striking demonstrations of the permanence of the associations of Hering's Law and also proofs that it is inborn and not learned. Helmholtz has only slight evidence that this association can be reduced artificially and then only to a minimal amount, but this is also true for many clearly inborn reflexes.

In chapter 28, *On pathology*, Hering, having established that his law is important with respect to the theory of disturbances of motility such as squint in myopes and hyperopes, now turns to deal with single muscle pareses.

For example, suppose that the left lateral rectus (LLR) has a mild paresis which produces double vision in the left visual field. We first consider the case of far vision. Increased tone to compensate for the weakness will develop in both lateral recti and will produce single vision. A hyperope, who uses positive accommodation with parallel lines of sight, then will also experience blur and must then give up either single vision or clear vision. If the subject is myopic, the increased innervation to both lateral recti will be helpful.

Next, Hering takes up the near vision case. As an emmetrope looks leftward the LLR is 'behind' the RMR and therefore needs less innervation to the adductors for convergence. There is therefore less positive accommodation and the patient needs to exert some accommodative effort. At first this will be all right, but if the demand becomes greater he has to give up either clear or single vision. For a patient who is also hyperopic this becomes more severe; if the patient is myopic, he is somewhat compensated already.

Thus we see that the hyperope is more sensitive to LLR paresis and may need to use strong convex lenses. The emmetrope is less sensitive and weak convex lenses may help. The myope may paradoxically be better off than he was without paresis. The area of double vision will be different in these three cases even though the paresis may be equal. Hering thus shows the excursion ability for LLR paresis to be worst for near vision and for hyperopia. Conversely, with medial rectus paresis everything is the opposite. All of these phenomena follow directly from Hering's Law.

Hering states that with asymmetrical convergence, it was thought that the medial rectus of the fixated eye was not innervated and also that there was no double innervation; the contrary is predicted by Hering's Law. Again, unequal innervation had been assumed for pathological cases, though we see that only a conceivable, but certainly not a large dissociation of central innate linking may occur. He generalizes the above to urge consideration of the distribution of balance between the medial and lateral recti when operative intervention is used, and he emphasizes the potential benefits of concave and convex glasses in these cases.

Summary of the Modern Status of Hering's Law

Introduction

1. Equal innervation is an important part of Hering's Law. The best modern reading of this is in terms of constraints on neurological control.
2. The law depends on simplicity. There exists a fixed pattern of innervation control, not altered either easily or to any considerable degree by learning, and not changed for different operating conditions such as initial position of the eye before a movement.
3. The law is an innate law and depends upon mechanisms incorporated into the 'hardwired' aspects of the brain through evolutionary selection.
4. The motor law has its counterpart in sensory function. The horizontal, vertical, and vergence degrees of freedom are important primarily for the sensory system and secondarily for the motor system.

The Single Eye

1. The same innervation ratio occurs in horizontal and vertical muscles for parallel movements independent of the initial position.
2. The vertical muscles act as one unit. The vertical recti and the oblique muscles summate so that the locus plane of the axes of vertical rotations is Listing's plane.
3. The horizontal and vertical planes of action are perpendicular to the line of sight and therefore have no first order effect on cyclorotation.
4. It is important to distinguish false torsion from true cyclorotation, and to distinguish the values of C_H from true cyclorotation. Helmholtz created a table of those values of C_H, for various horizontal and vertical directions of gaze, for which $C_L = 0$; that is, for which there is no true cyclorotation.
5. The simplicity of the law of constraint and the parallelism of movements with the same innervation ratios from different initial positions depends on two structural mechanical factors. These are the broad insertions of the tendons, and the fact that having four vertical muscles greatly widens the range of the vertical rotation forces.
6. As a consequence, Listing's Law is true within the smaller fixation space.
7. As a further consequence of the simplicity of the law of innerva-

tion, Donder's Law is true both within the smaller fixation space and at more extreme positions.

The Double Eye

1. Equal innervation goes to corresponding muscles.
2. The vertical muscles are treated as a single group and thus the correspondence between the two eyes is automatic for versional-vertical rotations.
3. Disjunctive correspondence must be accepted within the framework of application of the law to horizontal-vergence movements.
4. Hering mistakenly thought that vertical vergences were not natural, only made small deviations, and should be considered violations of Hering's Law. However, they are natural in that they compensate for disruptions for binocular co-linearity following vestibular-ocular compensation for head tilt. They can be large. Hering's Law can be analogously extended, as for horizontal-vergence, to include them.
5. If we proceed from the initial elegant consideration of Hering's Law for (i) horizontal versional movements to include (ii) vertical versional movements by treating the vertical muscles as a single motor, then add (iii) horizontal vergence by defining disjunctive correspondences, then append (iv) vertical vergences in an analogous fashion, and finally include (v) cyclorotational versions and (vi) cyclorotational vergences, we arrive at a point where Hering's Law appears to be tautological. Then, Hering's Law may be stated in terms of corresponding *movements* of the two eyes. Innervation is then that appropriate to the 'equal' eye movements. Indeed, both Hering, in 1879, and the texts of Duke-Elder and of Davson state Hering's Law in this tautological form.

Dynamics

Hering and Helmholtz scarcely made any dynamical observations. We now know dynamic violations of Hering's Law to be common. Indeed, these open the way for a better understanding of the 'hyperfine structure' of eye movements.

References

1. Berthold, *Archiv für Ophthalmologie, Vol. 11/13,* p. 107.
2. Burkhard, *Poggendorff's Annalen der Physik, Vol. 112,* 1861, p. 596.
3. Donders, *Holland. Beiträge zu d. Anat. u. Physiol. Wissenschaften, Vol. 1,* 1846.
4. Donders, *Ibid.,* p. 379.
5. Donders, *Die Anomalien der Refraction und Accommodation,* 1866.
6. Donders, *Ibid.,* p. 484.
7. Fick, *Zeitschrift f. Ration. Medicin, Vol. 4,* p. 801.
8. Helmholtz, H., *Verhandlungen des Heidelberger medicinisch naturhistorischen Vereines,* May 8, 1863.
9. Helmholtz, H., *Archiv für Ophthalmologie, Vol. 9/2,* p. 153.
10. Helmholtz, H., *Ibid.,* p. 189.
11. Helmholtz, H., *Physiologische Optik,* 1867, p. 471.
12. Helmholtz, H., *Ibid.,* p. 472.
13. Helmholtz, H., *Ibid.,* p. 473.
14. Helmholtz, H., *Ibid.,* p. 474.
15. Helmholtz, H., *Ibid.,* p. 519.
16. Helmholtz, H., *Ibid.,* p. 522.
17. Hering, E., *Beiträge zur Physiologie, Vol. 3,* 1863.
18. Hering, E., *Beiträge zur Physiologie, Vol. 3,* 1863, and *Vol. 4,* 1864.
19. Hering, E., *Archiv f. Anat. u. Physiol.* 1865, p. 164.
20. Listing, *Lehrbuch der Ophthalmologie von Reute,* p. 14.
21. MacGillavry, *Onderzoekingen over de Hoegrootheid der Accommodatie,* 1858.
22. Meissner, *Archiv für Ophthalmologie, Vol. 2,* pp. 1-123.
23. Meissner, *Beiträge zur Physiologie des Sehorganes.*
24. Müller, J., *Handbuch der Physiologie, Vol. 2,* 1840, p. 103.
25. von Recklinghausen, *Archiv für Ophthalmologie, Vol. 5/2,* p. 143.
26. Reute, *Ein Neues Ophthalmotrop,* p. 8.
27. Volkmann, *Neue Beiträge zur Physiologie des Gesichtsinnes,* 1836, p. 148.
28. Weber, E.H., *Programmata collecta. Summa doctrinae de motu iridis,* 182.
29. Wundt, W., *Archiv für Ophthalmologie, Vol. 8/2,* p. 1.

References for Introduction and Commentaries

Alpern, M. Movements of the Eyes. In Davson, H. (Ed.), *The Eye,* 3-187. New York: Academic Press, 1962.

Blakemore, C. Environmental Constraints on Development in the Visual System. In R. Hinde & J. Stevenson-Hinde (Eds.), *Constraints on Learning,* 51-74. London: Academic Press, 1973.

Bahill, A.T., Ciuffreda, K.J., Kenyon, R.V., & Stark, L. Dynamic and static violations of Hering's law of equal innervation. *Am. J. Opt.*, in press, 1976.

Bahill, A.T. & Stark, L. Neurological control of horizontal and vertical components of oblique saccadic eye movements. *Mathematical Biosciences 27,* 287-298, 1975.

Bahill, A.T. & Stark, L. Dynamic and static violations of Hering's Law of equal innervation. *American Journal of Optometry and Physiological Optics 53,* 798-808, 1976.

Boring, E. *A History of Experimental Psychology.* New York: Appleton-Century-Crofts, 1950.

Brecher, G. Die optokinetische Auslösung von Augenrollung und rotatorischem Nystagmus. *Arch. ges. Physiol. 234,* 13-28, 1934.

Coleman, W. *Biology in the Nineteenth Century: Problems of Form, Function, and Transformation.* New York: Wiley & Sons, 1971.

Cranefield, P. The organic physics of 1847 and the biophysics of today. *J. History of Med. 12,* 407-423, 1957.

Davson, H. *The Physiology of the Eye* (3rd edition). New York: Academic Press, 1972.

DeValois, R. & Jones, A. Single cell analysis of the organization of the primate color-vision system. In R. Jung & H. Kornhuber (Eds.), *The Visual System: Neurophysiology and Psychophysics.* Berlin: Springer-Verlag, 1961.

Duke-Elder, S. & Wybar, K. *System of Ophthalmology.* Volume 6: Ocular Motility and Strabismus. London: Henry Kimpton, 1973.

Elias, H. The liver cord concept after 100 years. *Science 110,* 470-472, 1949.

Garten, S. Ewald Hering zum Gedächtnis. *Arch. ges. Physiol. 170,* 501-522, 1918.

Helmholtz, H. *Physiologische Optik.* Leipzig: Voss, 1867.

Helmholtz, H. *Physiological Optics.* Transl. by Southall, J.P.C., 1925: Reissued by Dover Press, New York, 1962.

Hering, E. *Beiträge zur Physiologie.* Leipzig: W. Engelmann, 1861-1864.

Hering, E. *Die Lehre vom Binokularen Sehen.* Leipzig: W. Engelmann, 1868(a).

Hering, E. Die Selbststeuerung der Atmung durch den Nervus vagus. Nach Versuchen von Breuer. *Sitzber. d. k. k. Akad d. Wiss. zu Wien 57,* 672, 1868(b).

Hering, E. *Über das Gedächtnis als eine allgemeine Funktion der organisierten Materie.* Vienna: C. Gerold's Sohn, 1870.

Hering, E. *Zur Lehre vom Lichtsinn.* Vienna: C. Gerold's Sohn, 1878.

Hering, E. *Der Raumsinn und die Bewegungen des Auges.* in L. Hermann (Ed.), *Handbuch der Physiologie,* 3(1). Leipzig: F. Vogel, 1879. Transl. as *Spatial Sense and Movements of the Eye,* by C. Radde. Baltimore: Am. Acad. Optom., 1942.

Hering, E. Erklärung der Farbenblindheit aus der Theorie der Gegenfarben. *Lotos 1,* 13, 1880.

Hering, E. Über die spezifischen Energien des Nervensystems. *Lotos 5,* 116, 1884.

Hering, E. *Grundzüge der Lehre vom Lichtsinn.* Berlin: Springer, 1920. Transl. as *Outlines of a Theory of the Light Sense* by L. Hurvich & D. Jameson. Cambridge: Harvard U. Press, 1964.

Hering, E. & Sherrington, C. Über Hemmung der Kontraction willkürlicher Muskeln bei elektrische Reizung der Grosshirnrinde. *Arch. ges. Physiol. 68,* 222-228, 1897.

Hoffman, F. & Bielschowsky, A. Über die der Willkür entzogenen Fusionsbewegungen der Augen. *Arch. ges. Physiol. 80,* 1-40, 1900.

Hurvich, L. Hering and the scientific establishment. *Am. Psychologist 24,* 497-514, 1969.

Kertesz, A. The effect of stimulus complexity on human cyclofusional response. *Vision Res. 12,* 699-704, 1972.

Kertesz, A. & Jones, R. Human cyclofusional response. *Vision Res. 10,* 891-896, 1970.

Ogle, K. *Researches in Binocular Vision.* New York: Hafner, 1964.

Pribram, K. & Bridgeman, B. Retinally-oriented vs. environmentally-oriented modification of early visual environment. In prep.

Stark, L. *Neurological Control Systems: Studies in Bioengineering.* New York: Plenum Press, 1968.

Svaetichin, G. Spectral response curves from single cones. *Acta Physiol. Scand. 39,* Supp. 134, 17-46, 1956.

Ullman, E. About Hering and Breuer. In R. Porter (Ed.), *Breathing: Hering-Breuer Centenary Symposium.* London: J. & A. Churchill, 1970.

Verhoeff, F. Cycloduction. *Tr. Am. Ophth. Soc. 32,* 208-228, 1934.

Wundt, W. Über die Bewegung der Augen. *Arch. f. Ophth. 8,* 1-78, 1862.

Index